AF322573

Dr. Slaton Live™
Reflective Storytelling
The Crisis of Self!

Dr. Slaton Live™
Reflective Storytelling
The Crisis of Self!

*Understanding Brain, Body,
and Sense Messaging*

Christopher K. Slaton

Library of Congress Control Number: 2024923283

ISBN: 979-8-89228-334-2   (Paperback)
ISBN: 979-8-89228-335-9   (Hardcover)
ISBN: 979-8-89228-336-6   (eBook)

Printed in the United States of America

I want to extend my deepest gratitude to my daughter, Charmaine. Through her life, I became more attuned to the complexities of personal identity and "the crisis of self." Raising a child with special needs taught me how to engage with her unique experiences, particularly in addressing the challenges of sensory processing and communication difficulties. This journey allowed me to directly assess and work through what I now refer to as "sense path" and "receive path" obstacles. These terms helped guide my understanding of how to navigate and support her development.

Likewise, my son's life profoundly shaped who I am today. His battles with schizophrenia opened my eyes to the importance of learning to live, think, and respond together. We developed a deep, mutual understanding as we navigated both his mental health and our emotional well-being. Together, we learned how to provide physical, mental, and emotional care, and how to help each other move forward through life's challenges.

Without these experiences, I would not have developed the same sensitivity and awareness toward these vital areas of growth.

TABLE OF CONTENTS

WHY DR. SLATON LIVE™ IS THE VOICE OF BRAIN TALK

My son, Chris, used to say: "Speak the truth! My brain must lead my body through my sense of feel for self." This powerful message became my guide, helping me understand how critical it is to listen to our inner voice. Growing up in Oakland, I spent much of my time reflecting on my experiences, asking myself deep questions—did I want to be an athlete, a gang leader, or both? My inner voice helped me navigate my environment, interpreting people and situations in a way that led me to live authentically, even when I faced inner conflict.

Without my father around, I developed a poor attitude that influenced my behavior, though not my character. My inner voice became my compass, helping me recognize my feelings, body language, and states of mind. It moved me through phases of resistance—sometimes, I only cared about sex, sports, and gang activity. But despite my actions, I could always sense a pull toward doing the right thing, even while I was making poor decisions.

This inner voice became a crucial part of how I assessed myself. I realized that I was in crisis, that I needed to show more care, or I would face severe consequences, like getting locked up. Over time, as I began to care more for myself, others, and my environment, I felt my emotional pain lifting.

I could see how my physical responses—body language, posture, movement—were reflections of my inner self. I learned to interpret these signs as part of my behavior.

I became aware that the connection between my body and brain was key to understanding myself and the changes happening within me. Listening to my inner voice grounded me in self-care. It was a struggle, but I came to realize that I deeply cared about how I responded to my emotions, not just through thought, but in action. My inner voice gave me the strength and courage to accept self-criticism, and in that process, I discovered proof of my own consciousness.

By studying my body, behavior, and mind, I gained clarity: I was real, and what I did mattered to me. This realization formed the foundation of my understanding of human systems science, where the connection between the brain and the body helps us make sense of ourselves.

The way my brain interacts with my body through my senses informs me about my sense of self. This connection, which I call my "receive path," acts as a system of internal messaging. The choices I make—whether or not to listen to my inner voice—determine how effectively I can respond with care. I discovered that when my body led instead of my brain, I felt disconnected. My inner voice became more reactive, driven by external factors like social contact or the environment. It was as if my brain was offline, and I couldn't fully recognize the impact of my actions, including the harm I was causing others and myself.

To stop this cycle of aggression, I had to confront the uncomfortable emotions and rigid thoughts blocking my ability to reflect and connect. I realized that fear—fear of acknowledging the consequences—was holding me back. Tough guys aren't supposed to care, right? But this mindset kept me trapped, with my sense of self driving my physical reactions in a destructive loop.

As I began to change, I noticed a shift. My inner voice, which I now associate with "brain talk," became stronger. I started to feel my sense of self aligning with my brain's leadership. Though it was uncomfortable, the benefits of connecting my thoughts and emotions with my brain were undeniable. I realized that responding with care in moments of crisis was not a sign of weakness, but a strength. I learned to feel my way through interactions, using my inner voice to calm myself and improve my responses.

The process required me to get out of my own way—both my sense of self and my fear of the unknown. When I allowed my brain to lead, my inner voice guided me through decisions with greater clarity. "Brain talk" is the result of my receive path functioning properly: it processes the energy of my thoughts, body, and sensory input, all while enabling me to choose how I participate in my experiences. This choice, in turn, fosters self-learning.

For me, mental health has always been a challenge, but my inner voice became a vital tool in navigating emotions and thoughts. It taught me to assess feelings as emotional states (affect) and thoughts as cognitive processes (effect). Through this awareness, I developed my understanding of the sense and receive paths. States of mind, reflected through body language, belong to the "sense path," while reflection and thought arise from the "receive path." Learning to balance my external and internal sense of self has helped me show care and support for myself and others.

INTRODUCTION

I vividly recall sitting in my parents' living room as a child in the 1950s, watching television when the screen suddenly turned to static, and the noise from the TV startled me. Tension filled the room. We had just witnessed something unsettling—something that signaled something terrible had happened to the president. It was the day John F. Kennedy was assassinated, right there on the screen. At the time, I didn't fully understand the significance, but I could feel the weight of the moment. I can't explain why I cared, only that I did. My father's reaction—his visible concern—was enough to show me that this event mattered.

Just a few days earlier, my father had taken me with him to the repair shop. I remember watching as he argued with a white mechanic over the cost to fix our station wagon. This scene of everyday tension reflected much of the unspoken strain that surrounded my childhood.

I also remember my mother, who worked for the City of Emeryville in social work, allowing me to wait in the car as she handled her cases. These memories stand out, especially because my mother was recovering from a stroke and was still working through family issues. What I didn't know then was that my older brother had already turned to the streets, influenced by his peers and our grandmother. It wasn't until many years later, shortly before her passing in 2021, that my mother shared the full story with me. My brother had become a drug addict, and his struggles deeply affected her marriage to my father. This conversation gave me new insight into the pain my family had endured.

My mother had been reflecting on my 2016 book, *Education and Science: In the Best Interest of the Child*—a human systems research investigation addressing children from families affected by substance abuse. As she shared more details, I realized I had only scratched the surface of my brother's crisis. Through these conversations, I came to understand why I care so deeply about children and families in crisis. I had grown up witnessing, and feeling, the effects of a family torn apart by substance abuse and unresolved pain.

As the youngest of four boys and three girls, with one sister younger than me, I was surrounded by confusion and emotional disconnects. My parents and grandmother rarely communicated about the problems we were facing. However, my mother's revelations helped fill in those blanks. I had lived through my brother's struggles, his wife's heartache, and his children's pain, absorbing it all as if it were my own.

I often reflect on the conversations I had with my sister, Pam, who jokingly called me the "family social worker." It's within this context that I recall the signs of hurt, pain, and sadness I witnessed in my nieces and nephews as they grew up in crisis, unable to fully understand their emotions because of the love they still held for their parents. This is the heart of why I care so deeply about the work I do today.

This is why I created my own self-care learning practice, blending education and science to become a human learning consultant. I couldn't bear watching my nieces and nephews fall behind in school, nor could I stand the stress of seeing my siblings struggle with their own crises of self while ignoring my efforts to help them make meaningful changes in their environments—changes like the ones my mother had made for us. I felt the pressure to take action, to do something constructive that might inspire them to follow my lead.

So, my wife and I began setting goals and objectives to study this "crisis of self" more deeply. She became my first student of *Progressive Investing,* a framework we developed together. From this partnership, we crafted an action-learning theory: *learning how to live each day to become more informed.* We understood that achieving these goals required a blend of higher education to address the complexities of personal crises and scientific inquiry to comprehend the spread of pain, hurt, and sadness.

This led me to design **Human Systems Research.** I knew I needed to remove my own pain, hurt, and sadness from the equation to effectively help others. This research begins with the study of oneself in relation to others and the environment. The key is to clear your mind of any assumptions about the people you're working with—whether they are clients, participants, or even loved ones. The goal is to let their information flow freely into your "sense path," free from the tension, stress, or pressure to respond from your own perspective. The environment must be set up with signs of care, creating a space where they can engage through "brain talk"—a process that begins with introspection and evolves into meaningful social dialogue.

This journey led to the development of **Human Systems Science**, which focuses on the study of the brain, body, and sensory systems in relation to how we process information.

It became clear to me that understanding the flow of information—whether it's emotional, physical, or mental—was critical in helping people overcome the challenges caused by major life events. I began working with parents and children in crisis, observing how they made contact with one another and how they engaged in moments of interaction. I could see whether they accepted or rejected help, whether they participated or held back, and how their sense and receive path transformations—how they processed energy, actions, and feelings—played out in real-time.

This journey led to the development of **Feeling Systems Science**, which focuses on studying how individuals with sense and receive path problems experience and process their feelings. The key distinction emerged between a *sense of self* and a *sense of feel for self*, which reflects the brain-body connection influenced by social, cognitive, and environmental factors. Through this lens, we explore how the body and brain interact—where contact must be felt and transformed through a *sense of feel for self*, connecting brain and body in meaningful ways.

Feeling Systems Science allows us to study how information flows through the body and brain, deepening our understanding of how the brain learns, the body lives, and the senses interpret experiences. This science became crucial in our work with families in crisis, particularly with children born to parents who had abused drugs during pregnancy. Through this work, we began observing the concept of disconnection between sense and receive path functions, which manifested in various ways within these families.

This book introduces critical concepts:

- **Contact as the life source of the body**
- **Interaction as the learning source of the brain**
- **Cooperation as the thinking source of the senses**
- **Participation** as the response to feelings of emotion and thought within the sense path
- **Performance** as the forward and backward feedback loop that connects brain and body, shaping both a sense of self and a sense of feel for the brain in control of the body.

From these foundational ideas, we arrived at the concept of **Brain Talk**, which gave rise to the *Dr. Slaton Live™* series—focusing on how the brain processes information through self-talk and brain talk. This expanded the dialogue about how the brain senses and receives information. These ideas culminated in my 2012 book, where I explore **mentation**—the art and science of thinking—through contact and interaction. In this work, I examine how self-talk and brain talk function as core principles of action learning.

The book, *Education and Science: Save Our Youth*, emphasizes the importance of community-based learning to improve California's public schools. It highlights strategies for helping children, youths, and young adults, as well as providing resources for parents, teachers, and human-service professionals. This book also features the *Dr. Slaton Live™* series and showcases the **2011-2012 Pilot Merced Building Human Assets Project**, where these principles were put into practice.

I am Dr. Christopher Kevin Slaton, performing as *Dr. Slaton Live™*—the Ultimate Experience, the Brain's Body, and the Voice of Brain Talk. My mission is to write to the brain by investing in child development through **sense and receive path research**, aiming to improve the understanding of social and academic transformations of self.

The way I write about individuals—both self and others—within the contexts of home, school, neighborhood, and workplace networks is to guide family leaders in shaping their approach to developing a family as a business. This is why I emphasize teaching through the conceptualization of **community-based learning**.

A community is more than just a location—it is a place to practice living, learning, thinking, and responding to social contact and environmental influences. By focusing on these aspects, we can combat the pain, hurt, and sadness that often contribute to family decline.

PART ONE

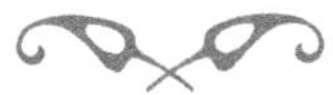

I feel like a **Brain Talker**. *My sense of feel for both my brain and body forms my understanding of self. The connection between my body and brain drives the flow of energy, actions, and emotions. Neural interactions between the two create a dynamic loop, where sense and receive path functions work together. My senses link the physical aspects of my body to the neuro-physical processes of my brain, forming a system of messaging.*

In other words, I describe the brain, body, and senses as the core information processing tools of my **Brain's Body**. *My body acts as a physical, social, and external influence, shaping my self-contact. Meanwhile, my brain serves as the neuro, mental, and emotional center, guiding my self-interactions. The senses, through the exchange of energy, actions, and feelings, are what allow me to make informed choices and engage cooperatively with the world around me.*

1. Your Brain is the Lead Social Organ.

Ever wonder why it is important to understand how contact influences the way you interact? In **human systems science**, the interaction between your brain, body, and senses is key. This relationship forms the foundation of mental, physical, and environmental contact, creating process loops that help you become more informed. By exploring how these elements influence one another, you gain a deeper understanding of how your interactions shape your responses and development.

Progressive Investing Model 1

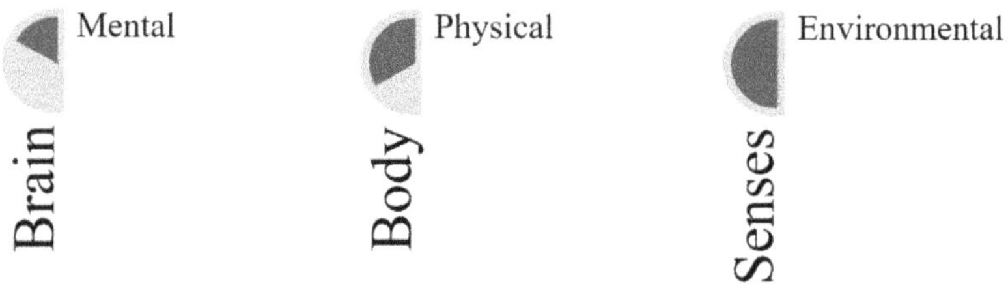

The reason we can engage in this dialogue is that your brain, body, and sense organs form a communication system that enables interaction. But before we dive into how we interact, we must first consider **sense contact** as the foundation of self-awareness—what I call the **physics of self**. This is how we evolve through our external sense of self. This is why I practice **human systems science**: it allows me to address the body as an external influence that shapes how I look, act, and experience feelings. The moment I begin to interact with my body to make sense of it, I create a **process loop**—the intersection between my *sense of self* and my *sense of feel for self*. My brain actively reads and assesses my body, creating a social and environmental understanding of self.

Through this, my **inner voice** emerges, as I develop a sense of myself based on physical observations that my brain reads and interprets. This transformation moves from an external *sense of self* to an internal *sense of feel for self*—a shift that is processed and refined by the brain. These connections will be explored throughout this book. In other words, my inner voice speaks through my internal sense of self, which is influenced by my experiences with the outer world. My brain, body, and senses are constantly transmitting messages. This is why human systems science is a game-changer—it focuses on the **receive path**, which enables me to process and respond to how my brain and body interact with the world.

My subjective *sense of feel for self* creates a feedback loop for my inner voice, guiding how I choose the best path to respond. This is where **sense and receive path research** comes into play—the study of my body as a physical experience and my self as a neuro-physical experience. Conflicts, or **crises of self**, arise during the transformation between body-mind influences and brain-body connections. I study the brain to understand the body, and I study both to learn about the senses—the **neuro-physics** of the Brain's Body. In this framework, the brain takes the lead, as we learn to manage the flow of energy and emotion, action and thought, and feelings and reflection by practicing sense and receive path research.

This is **brain talk**—the process of responding using your natural sense and receive systems. When you engage in brain talk, you are not only self-reporting but also creating new ways to express personal growth through self-leadership. Your brain responds through forward feed, communicating back to you via the way you sense and feel the words you read, the things you write, the images you create, and the actions you take to realize your experiences. It also includes how you perform, showcasing your talents and expressing yourself through noises, sounds, signs, and symbols. This process brings your brain talk into the physical world.

Your inner voice constantly processes social and emotional information for self-analysis, but when you bring these internal processes into the public realm, it becomes brain talk. When you are comfortable with the transformations between your *sense of self* and your *sense of feel for self*—through how you choose to receive and respond to both negative and positive contact—you are fully engaging in this process.

This dialogue is possible because of your brain's **self-healing system**. Recovering from damages to your ability to sense and receive social contact and neuro interaction requires the practice of **sense and receive path research**. This approach helps you understand how your brain functions as a feeling system, how your body acts as a physical environment, and how your senses work as social, neuro, and physical systems that rely on self-care experiences. It's an error to look only outward without also looking inward to understand how to live with yourself, learn with yourself, think with yourself, and respond with your brain in the lead. Without this, conflict arises—a **crisis of self**.

In **human systems science**, *learning* means that your brain is the experience through your *sense of feel for self*—a key function of the receive path. *Living* refers to your body as the contact point through which your *sense of self* traverses, guided by sense path transfers. The brain and body are interconnected: when the brain leads, it transforms the receive path functions. Once the brain establishes this connection to the body, the goal is to learn how to live through both positive and negative experiences of contact and interaction. These experiences create forward and backward exchanges between states of mind and feelings of thought.

The backward feed reflects the body's behavior, while the forward feed is the brain's response. This dynamic can influence whether your inner voice leads to conflict or peace, generating tension, stress, or pressure—or, alternatively, allowing you to choose how to respond thoughtfully rather than react impulsively.

The body reacts to live, while the brain responds to learn how to live through the process of backward and forward self-analysis. This distinction between your **inner voice** and **brain talk** is crucial. Your inner voice triggers body-mind interactions, allowing you to reflect on social and environmental influences. However, **brain talk** goes beyond introspection. It engages the **receive path functions**, which influence your *sense of feel for self* and allow the brain to respond with thought, reflection, and emotion in control of the body.

This distinction explains why you can recover from poor choices and decisions over time, improving how you learn to live, learn to learn, learn to think, and learn to respond. The connection between your brain and body functions as a **sense and receive technology**—constantly evolving your sense of self to meet the internal needs of your sense of feel for self. As these connections develop, the neuro-physics of the Brain's Body become fully realized, allowing you to navigate life more effectively.

2. This Conversation Applies to Brain Talk and the Brain's Body.

The way your brain interacts with your body and your senses is to learn, live, feel and think through the experience of self. But ask yourself: Can you learn without a *sense of feel* for your brain? Can you live without a *sense of feel* for your body? Can you think without a *sense of feel* for your senses?

A core concept of this book is that **Brain Talk** represents a telepathic exchange of energy between your *sense of feel for your brain* and the **neuro-physics of self**—what I call your **Brain's Body.** This connection is what allows you to navigate the complexities of life with greater awareness and control.

Progressive Investing Model 2

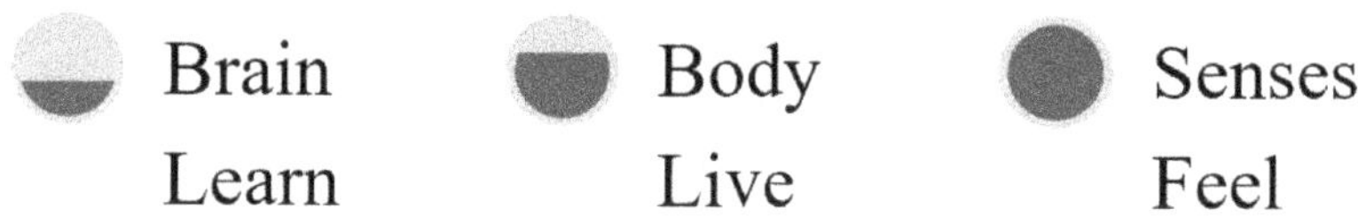

Human Systems Science is about learning how the brain learns, how the body lives, and how the senses feel things. I write about the **crisis of self** as a learning crisis, where the messages we receive from contact and interaction affect, influence, or alter how the brain learns, how the body lives, and how the senses feel. This involves the brain sending information forward, the body sending information backward, and the senses receiving and sending information both ways—reacting instead of responding. These are the physical and neuro transformations that shape **brain talk**, **body language**, and **inner voice exchanges**, leading to struggles between a *sense of self* and a *sense of feel for self.*

It is your choice to practice using the language introduced throughout this book, designed to help you navigate the crisis of self and the changes that occur in your encoded states of mind. For instance, *forward and backward feed* refers to how you comprehend the ways in which contact challenges you through interaction. Often, the way you use your body to live can be at odds with how your brain processes learning. To resolve this tension, I guide you through **sense and receive path research**, which helps decode your *sense of self*—the observable, external you—and your *sense of feel for self*—the invisible neuro-processes occurring internally.

This tension reflects the back-and-forth struggle between body contact and brain interaction, influenced by emotion and thought. The **receive path** is highly susceptible to the effects of social contact and environmental factors, which means your brain's neuro response sends forward emotions and reflective thoughts. This creates a **backward feed** from your body-mind connection (the observable experience) and a **forward feed** from your brain-body connection (the neuro-physical response). Confusion can arise between the physical self and the neuro-physical self—where backward feed from the **sense path** conflicts with forward feed from the **receive path**.

This is where your **inner voice** might struggle to focus the flow of information between your *sense of self* and *sense of feel for self.* This connection is essential to help you transition from **body-mind** influences to **brain-body** influences, allowing you to live through the experience of self and learn through the experience of self and the brain as points of transformation. This is a unique type of self-learning—one where you seek to understand the **physics** behind your self-esteem and the **neuro-physics** behind your self-doubt by studying your brain, body, and sense events. You begin to explore **brain talk**, **body language**, and the processes of **sense and receive path conversion**. Your inner voice operates between the influences of your *sense of self, sense of feel for self*, and the brain, continually testing your brain-body connections.

The **crisis of self** emerges when you struggle to move through contact and interaction, specifically in how you choose to sense and receive negative or positive information. Your body experiences contact, while your brain processes these exchanges as a forward-and-backward struggle to live and learn simultaneously. Feedback from your inner voice signals that something is off, causing you to withdraw from participating in the connection between your *sense of feel for self* and your brain's role in leading the body. When this withdrawal happens, the resulting pain, hurt, and sadness manifest as anger, fear, anxiety, frustration, disappointment, or even hostility. These emotions trap you in states of mind that make it difficult to adjust to the transitions between **sense** and **receive path** functions.

When emotion and thought flow backward from contact, it indicates that you've rejected the choice to fully engage in the experience. There is less motivation to transfer the experience into learning how it feels to participate in the **sense and receive path interplay** between brain, body, and sense messaging. Pain disrupts the flow of energy, hurt impedes action, and sadness influences feelings. This withdrawal isolates your *sense of self* from your *sense of feel for self* and the brain. You begin to detach from the way it feels to interact without the physics of self or body language in the lead of brain activity. Instead, you react in ways that reduce forward feed and receive path cycles, seeking to appear calm or collected on the surface but avoiding genuine engagement.

To truly respond—with the brain in the lead of the body—you must embrace the **brain's body** connection. This involves remaining present in the experience, collecting your *sense of feel for self* and allowing the brain to lead the body, enabling you to respond rather than react.

The Conversion Process to Brain Talk involves moving beyond your *sense of self* and the programmed mind-body states triggered by external contact, which influences your receive path functions. This process allows you to consciously choose to accept the way you think before feeling how energy, action, and emotions move through the receive path. By doing this, your inner voice gains the power to organize the backward flow—transforming emotions into *feelings of thought* with reflection, enabling you to respond with managed emotions.

The role of your **sense of feel** is to process emotions and thoughts during social interactions via the sense path. With your brain in the lead, your inner voice facilitates learning how to respond cooperatively, allowing for meaningful engagement through thought and emotion, rather than reactive responses.

3. The Complex Exchanges between a Sense of Self with a Sense of Feel for Self.

When I say **sense**, I mean *contact*. When I say **receive**, I mean *interaction*. When I say **feel**, I mean *neuro experience*. Any sense contact with the body triggers a response, like an alarm. The challenge arises when you choose to ignore how you *feel* the contact, which can block the transformation process between your *sense of self* and your *sense of feel for* *self.* This can cause the body to react impulsively, affecting how the brain responds to external interactions.

In essence, your **sense and receive path interplay** functions as a process loop—how contact is sensed and received shapes the ongoing dynamic between body and brain.

Progressive Investing Model 3

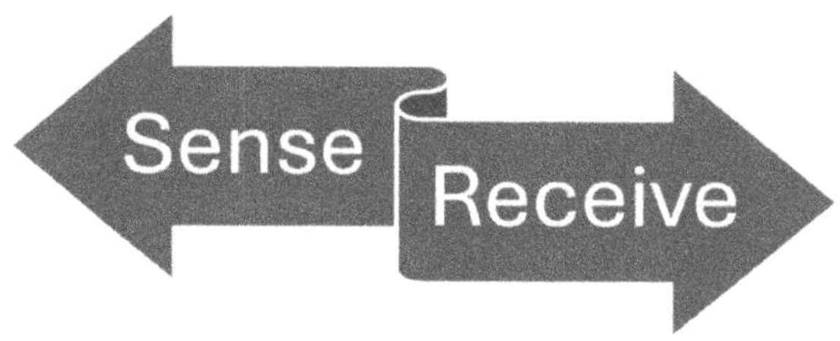

The **sense path** represents the behaviors of the body, while the **receive path** reflects the neuro responses of the brain. Your *sense of who you are* is expressed through how you use your body to communicate—your body language. When you sense self-contact, you enter a process loop that identifies the **physics of self**. As you sense and feel the physics of self, you engage in reciprocal exchanges or transformations of backward and forward feed—where the sense and receive paths interphase.

This is why focus plays a crucial role: it helps center your *sense of feel for self* on actions that allow you to experience your brain's activity. Through the **sense, feel, and focus process cycle**, you practice experiencing the **neuro physics of self**. This practice helps you understand how your body processes contact and how it influences your emotions, thoughts, and reflections as part of the dynamic interaction between sense and receive path functions.

Progressive Investing Model 4

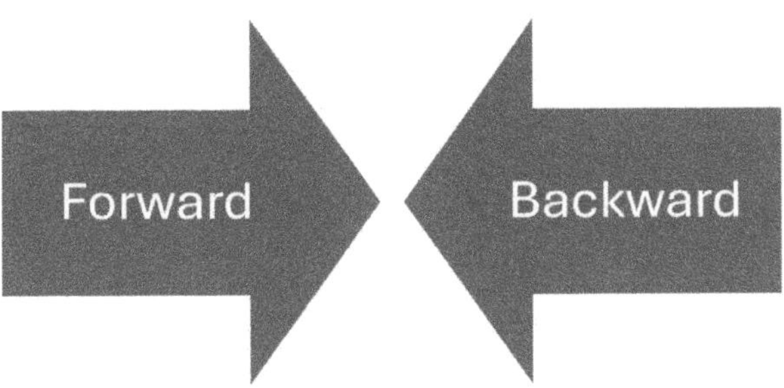

Your **sense of feel for self** evolves as the brain's neural systems interact with the physical systems of the body. The flow of energy, action, and feelings enables the transfer of emotions, thoughts, and reflections between the brain, body, and senses—forming a loop of forward and backward exchanges. These exchanges are processed through **sense and receive path conversion functions**, forming the foundation for **self-learning**, which acts as a catalyst to enhance brain-body connections.

The guiding principle here is that your sense of feel for self, with the brain leading the body, drives self-learning through the **neuro physics of self-research, self-discovery, and self-help**—all explored within the framework of **human systems science**.

Understanding the interplay between brain, body, and senses as a network requires a sense of feel for self, particularly regarding thought, reflection, and emotion, as these elements influence the forward feed of brain activity in response to contact. Interaction, therefore, extends from the **receive path**, which processes both negative and positive senses of self—be it social emotion, thought, or reflection. These, in turn, fuel the struggles between backward and forward feed in the **receive path**.

Cooperation between brain, body, and senses is essential for self-help. As neural activity occurs in the receive path, self-learning requires you to cooperate with the transfer process to your sense of feel for self, rather than resisting the feelings these transactions evoke about yourself, others, and the world.

When you are committed to **self-learning**—understanding how your brain learns, how your body lives, and how your senses feel—you will find it easier to navigate the struggle between self-identity and ego. As you learn to cooperate with your sense of feel for self and your brain's body, your learning loops expand, fostering deeper participation in a collective sense of feel for self, others, and the environment where contact and interaction occur.

This is why understanding your **sense and receive path action** requires a higher level of participation to fully integrate your sense of self with your sense of feel for self, with the brain leading the body. This is not typical action learning; it is about learning through contact and interaction, navigating the transformation between your sense of self and your sense of feel for self—requiring elevated cooperation to achieve true self-understanding.

In **human systems science**, **care** is a sign of your willingness to engage in the learning process of your brain, body, and senses. Care serves as a way to assess your performance, reflecting your commitment to personal growth. Every action you take to **learn how to live, learn, think, and respond** becomes a performance indicator that measures your levels of self-mastery—both forward and backward.

In the **physics of self-learning through reflection**, mastering yourself requires learning how to manage your brain, control your body, and focus your senses. This enables you to perform effectively in various environments, including home, school, neighborhood, and workplace networks. These performances rely on your ability to integrate **self-action**, the actions of others, and interactions with your environment.

When you live through a **sense of feel for self**, guided by the brain and expressed through signs of care, your *sense of self* is confronted with the consequences of resisting, ignoring, or denying the brain's role in leading the body.

4.　How Your Inner Voice Converts to Brain Talk.

As you begin to understand how brain, body, and sense messaging feels, the information flow between your *sense of self* and your *sense of feel for self* carries both the *affects of emotion* and the *effects of thought*, which I describe as your **inner voice**. But how do you experience your inner voice?

You might tense up, ball your hands into fists, stare me down, or twist and turn in your seat as if you want to lash out—but this is not the way to address your inner voice. I can feel your anger, sense your fear, and observe your anxiety through your body's reactions. When I use talk, I follow four key steps:

1. **Assess contact** as a sense act,
2. **Assess interaction** as a receive act,
3. **Assess cooperation** as a process act,
4. **Assess participation** as acts of care.

Though you can still hear me, it seems you lack the ability or desire to engage in the conversation. You weren't ready to receive my talk—my instruction.

Brain talk! I kept observing. You didn't take a breath to calm yourself. You didn't practice feeling your way through my contact or respond to my signs of care. You weren't truly *feeling* me. There were few signs of cooperation or willingness to work through your reactions. I saw no indication of thought or reflection that would help us move through the situation without further agitating your emotions. Your body language felt frozen, with no sign of response or forward movement.

As my brain, body, and sense connections continued to send feelings through my contact and interaction, my own **sense, feel, and focus process cycles** kept me centered in the loop. I could feel your pain, hurt, and sadness manifesting in your observable body-mind state, and my concern grew. My goal was to help you focus your anger, fear, and anxiety on my signs of care—long enough for you to sense my cooperation.

Your brain, body, and sense connections, or lack thereof, were evident. **Brain talk** happens at different levels: contact helps you live, interaction helps you learn, cooperation helps you think, and participation allows you to respond.

Progressive Investing Model 5

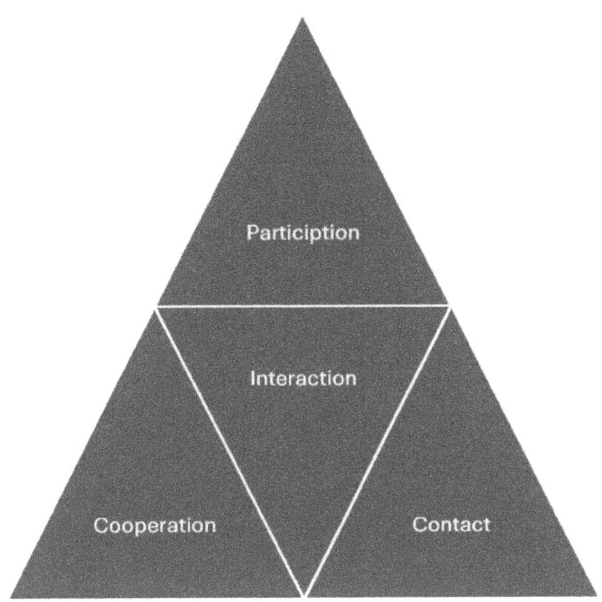

For more than 30 years, I have studied the **brain, body, and sense systems** of children and parents in crisis, those I have had the honor of working with in the development of **Human Systems Science**. This focus involves understanding the conversion processes between the *inner voice* and **brain talk**, analyzing how brain, body, and sense messaging operates. My journey began with a report in my 2006-2008 **Progressive Investment Reports**, which I submitted to California's federal, state, county, and local government leaders, as well as political and business figures. In these reports, I examined why all children may not be able to learn effectively.

I was investigating **substance abuse-related disorders** that impact parent-child bonding, which led me to study **sense and receive path research**—specifically, how parents and children communicate through body language, states of mind, and the inner voice that converts into **brain talk**. I discovered that many children fail to respond to a teacher's request for participation in the classroom because they expect the teacher to understand their inner dialogue without converting it into spoken words. This confusion stems from the difference between the informal use of talk at home and the structured use of language in school. Learning to use talk in the home supports the child's *inner voice development*, whereas learning to use language in school is more technical and suited to *brain talk*.

For instance, the inner voice you hear as you read this book responds to your external *sense of self*, sending **backward feed** to inform your *sense of feel for self* and your brain. Your brain then releases **forward feed**, synthesizing feelings of emotion and thought through reflection. This feedback loop is the product of brain, body, and sense interactions, functioning through **sense and receive path processes**.

In essence, the inner voice you hear is a reaction to social contact and environmental interaction. Your internal *sense of feel* reacts to these experiences, deciding whether to avoid or accept urges to cooperate. This cooperation determines whether you participate in the exchanges between your brain and body, where sense and receive path functions facilitate the flow of information.

In observing my students' bodies as they responded to instructions to read, write, draw, or calculate, I could sense from the tension in their eyes and hand movements that something was wrong. Instead of engaging with the instruction, they would become more animated or withdraw into a physical state of resistance or defiance. This classroom setting served as a laboratory for studying children born to parents who may have abused drugs while in utero. The way their bodies reacted revealed a disconnect between brain and body cooperation. The body was leading the brain, as my contact and instructions were met with resistance, triggering emotional responses rather than thoughtful reflection. I recorded these responses as **states of mind**—defensive reactions reflecting a lack of forward thought.

When I use the term **state of mind**, I am referring to a defensive state of reflection, where the transfer of experience to the **receive path** is resisted or rejected, affecting the student's *sense of feel for self* and the brain. Instead of generating a **backward feed**, these students exhibited signs of withdrawal or isolation from my contact and interaction. This is why I chart signs of cooperation to assess their level of participation in the **sense and receive path exchanges** of energy, action, and feelings—both external and internal. A **state of mind** becomes a fixed response to contact. For example, a student's **safe sense of self** might manifest as anger at the point of contact, fear during interaction, and anxiety at the point of cooperation. I could feel my students resisting changes in their body language, holding tightly to their specific states of mind.

This response was often to the social environment, where the child reacted to the **physics of self** and their body as a defensive **mood state**. My goal was to understand what was happening and how the child's **inner voice** played a role. My objective was to contribute to our knowledge base on **sense and receive path research**, systematically assessing performance in response to these interactions. For instance, I assess:

1. **Contact** as sense data from the breath of life onward,

2. **Interaction** as a receive path impulse from the act of breathing,

3. **Cooperation** as a variable influenced by internal/external signs of care, and

4. **Participation** as a performance indicator between forward and backward feed in sense and receive path interplay.

In essence, a student's response to the social environment—including me—engages their capacity to sense and feel the **physics of self** as states of mind emanating from their **inner voice** through introspection.

A student may seek to live in their **body-mind** as an imaginary space, where they maintain contact with their *sense of self* as an objective behavior goal. However, the **body-mind conversion process** often conflicts with the transfer of inner dialogue to **brain-body connections**, where **brain talk** emerges from the sense of feel for contact, as a forward feed of thought and reflection. I refer to the conversion process for learners who may suffer from **sense and receive path damage**, which affects the link between their sense of self and sense of feel for self. The **inner voice** must convert into **brain talk**, which transfers from social contact as forward feed, resulting in thought with reflection.

Your **brain** communicates with your body through your *sense of feel for self.* The body, in turn, experiences social contact and environmental influences, which activate your **inner voice**. This inner voice emerges from your experiences of self, other people, and the environment, prompting you to respond. The initial response begins with introspection, or **self-talk**, which must then convert into **brain talk** through **backward feed** as you act in response to your environment through social interaction.

Social interaction generated by brain talk provides observable feedback, serving as clear proof of how well your **sense and receive path** functions are performing. In other words, **signs of care** serve as evidence of effective communication between your body-mind and brain-body, reflecting the success of the conversion process cycles.

5. Talk to your brain with signs of care.

Brain talk is the connection between your brain and body that helps you overcome reactions to contact, particularly when negative energy disrupts the flow. When your brain takes the lead, your **inner voice** engages through **signs of care**, allowing you to respond using **forward feed**. In contrast, when you rely solely on your *sense of feel for self*, you are often trying to regain control over your body's reactions.

Throughout my studies, I have worked with many parents, teachers, coaches, counselors, nurses, and other human services professionals who chose not to use **signs of care** when making contact through the **physics of self**, other people, and the environment. I observed that this often resulted in resistance from the individuals they were trying to engage, as their contact lacked the essential signs of care necessary for meaningful interaction.

These professionals failed to realize that they, as physical, mental, and emotional symbols, can be sensed and felt by others. When they did not convey signs of care, the people they interacted with—especially those in a **crisis of self**—perceived the absence of care. This perception blocked access to their **sense of feel for self** and the brain's leadership over the body. Without sufficient signs of care, the **inner voice** concludes that the interaction lacks the necessary support for connection and cooperation.

Progressive Investing Model 6

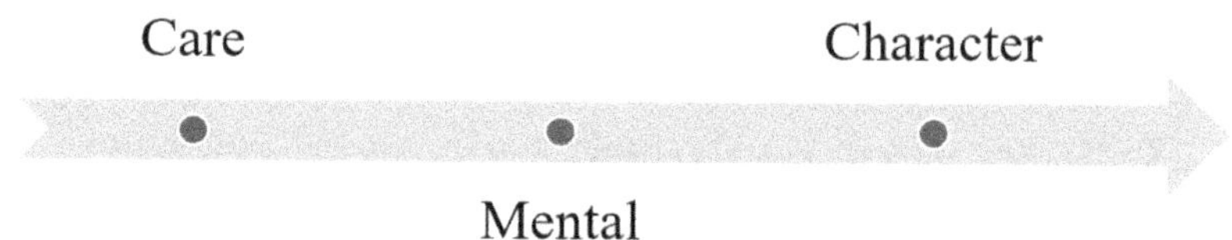

Care is a competitive challenge, determining whether you connect or disconnect your brain-body connections to resolve conflicts in your **sense and receive paths**. Instead of being overwhelmed by the emotional effects of negative thinking, you can focus on your *sense of feel for self* and engage your brain to take a more mental, thoughtful approach. The ultimate conflict lies in the tension between *who you are* and *what you are becoming* during the flow of information. In other words, do you have the knowledge to understand the experience? Does your social sense of self provide the strength to transfer feelings of fear, anger, or anxiety into the **receive path**? **Care** becomes a character struggle—the decision to choose the appropriate response.

You can sense or feel the internal tension, outer stress, and the neuro-physical energy and actions that form as signs of who you are or what you may become. This is when the **body-mind** takes control, often displayed through **body language** indicating withdrawal or avoidance, a **negative response** to contact. This state of mind, expressed as feelings through body language, must be overcome. When your sense path is disrupted, you need to adjust your body language, seeking ways to connect with the other person's *inner sense of feel* for your contact—especially when negative feelings from the past or present are involved.

Body language often signals: *Approach with caution and respect for my right to reject you as a negative influence on my self-reflection.* If your contact is perceived as negative, the person's body may reflect signs of anger or defensive behavior.

Care is essential for managing the flow of emotions, controlling thoughts, and processing sensory experiences. This **brain, body, and sense network** is integral to how you learn to live each day, informing, disciplining, and focusing yourself to respond thoughtfully to negative feelings. By engaging **signs of care** for yourself, others, and the environment, you use the **physics of the body** to ground your actions and the **neuro-physics of the brain** to stay in control.

The **conversion of self** as the brain's body must be carefully managed, controlled, and processed through both positive and negative sense and receive path functions. This process is essential to performing the mental feedback cycles that help clarify human learning goals and guide personal development.

You either **look** for signs of care or **feel** for them. **Character** is the social and mental quality that manifests in response to social contact or environmental interaction through the **neuro physics of self**. In the face of contact, your focus shifts as **social-cognitive interactions** move through your brain and body, allowing feelings of thought to emerge as reflections on the experience. Although this may seem precarious, each act is influenced by your temperament. You either feel comfortable with your sense of self, or you feel indifferent to the sensations of energy, action, and feelings moving through you—impulses that could make you more caring and thoughtful.

You might not be inherently good or bad, but a lack of care can impact how you make negative or positive contact with yourself, others, and the environment. Once you experience negative contact through your sense of self, you have a choice: do you let your actions reflect that negativity, or do you want to feel good by choosing a more positive path? Your **physical self** represents your *sense of self* and body, while your **mental self** embodies your *sense of feel* for your brain and body. When you choose to care about how you feel, you are cooperating with the experience of sensing and receiving social contact, participating in either negative or positive emotional and cognitive interactions.

When you care to learn how to live, the way you think about what you feel shapes your mental identity. You begin to appreciate the process of responding, becoming more aware of your character through these **signs of care**. This is the brain work of your **receive path functions**, which release **forward feed** in the form of thought, prompting reflective actions. You must accept the role that care plays in navigating negative or positive feelings toward yourself, others, and the environment, to fully experience how you sense, transfer, and receive thought with reflection.

This perspective is about **progressive investing**. **Self-motivation** becomes a process loop in which you live each day to become more informed, guided by signs of care for the experience of information processing.

Promoting **signs of care** works both ways: in how you **sense cognitive energy** and how you **receive cognitive action**. The **physics of self-growth** through care allows you to carry forward a sense of awareness, applying your social and emotional talents as needed to adapt to different situations.

Helping means caring enough to move beyond your negative sense of self. Your social-cognitive energy reflects your body and the **language of your states of mind**, feeding back into your behavior. If your **sense path** is blocked, it can hinder the feedback loop between your *sense of feel* for yourself, others, and the environment. In other words, your body language may not be releasing signs of thought and reflection as evidence of care, impacting your effectiveness as a helper.

6.   Do you feel me?

I am **progressively investing in Brain Talk**. Every word carries energy, action, and feelings, as each word expresses what it feels like to sense, feel, and focus your **brain-body connections**. When you lead through your *sense of feel for self* and your brain, you unlock new understandings through this incredible experience. Do you feel a sense of connection to my words?

This book is about moving beyond a simple *sense of self* to explore how poor responses to social contact and environmental influences can hinder your growth, making it harder to become more cooperative and participatory in processing emotions. This involves engaging with **feelings of thought and reflection**. I used to easily unravel when social contact triggered resistance in my inner voice because I didn't understand the natural interplay between self, others, and the environment.

That's why I apply a **Human Systems Research** approach throughout this book—to describe how it feels, or how it fails to feel, the connection between self, others, and the environment when **sense and receive path functions** are damaged.

Progressive Investing Model 7

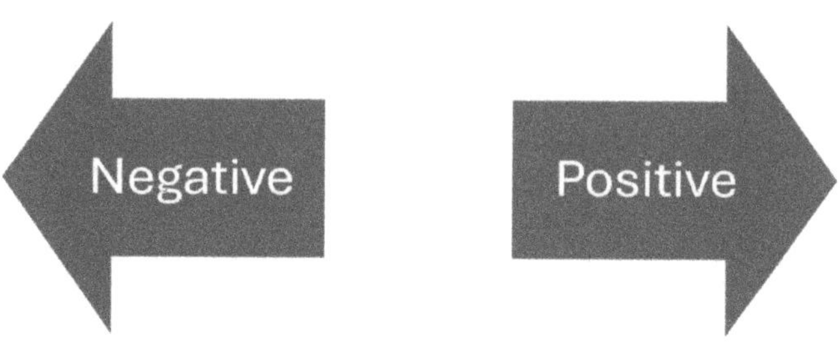

Negative refers to regressive energy, action, or feelings, while **positive** represents progressive energy, action, or feelings. This **progressive investing model** describes how information flow impacts your ability to learn how to live through the experience of self—through **brain, body, and sense messaging**. Can you sense and feel how your inner voice carries both negative and positive **forward and backward feed**? You feel your *sense of self* as the event, and your *sense of feel for self* as the goal, allowing you to assess how positive and negative information influences you.

Now, imagine not being able to feel for yourself, others, or the environment due to **sense path damage** caused by major life events. This would be like losing the ability to develop **feelings of thought and reflection**, preventing you from processing emotions. You might react by resisting social contact or withdrawing, as your **inner voice** urges you to isolate. This is the **intersection between sense and receive path functions**, which empower you to live, learn, think, and respond as a **human system**. Your brain allows you to feel because your body connects to it. The way social contact influences your emotions can affect the transfer to the **receive path process loops**.

The **receive path** powers your knowledge, helping you transition from a *sense of self* to a *sense of feel for self*—the formation of your inner voice, which expresses how it feels to experience brain, body, and sense action and emotions.

When you resist the flow of emotion in social contexts, you fail to participate in the transformation of self—from just sensing the experience to truly feeling it through brain, body, and sense coaction. **Receive path knowledge** includes how you transfer emotions through **forward feed**, triggering feelings of thought and reflection as **backward feed**. This flow happens when you practice engaging with feelings long enough for feedback to reshape how your sense and receive path functions interact.

Interaction transforms old energy, action, and feelings into new ways to sense the actions of the body and feel the processes of the brain. When you cooperate to learn through both positive and negative feelings, you develop **sustainable signs of self-help** through physical self-analysis. In other words, the **neuro-physics of self** is **brain talk**.

This is where you learn to shift into the **brain's body**. When my students adjust to my contact as an external influence, I can assess their **brain, body, and sense formatting**. Formatting refers to the way they display mental, physical, and social energy. They have moved beyond their *sense of self* and restructured their *sense of feel for me* as a **receive path influence**, allowing them to practice aligning brain, body, and sense coaction. I can sense the flow of information through their signs of **physical discipline**, reflected as feelings of cooperation. In this process, they accept my physical models of care and adjust the way they use talk to interact with their sense of feel for me.

A student practicing **progressive investing** creates their own learning style through self-discovery, working to release feelings of hurt, pain, or sadness for various reasons. My goal is to generate **positive feedback** in their inner voice, guiding them through **action learning** to release negative energy. This can be achieved through activities like reading, writing, drawing, acting, and performing, all expressed as **brain talk**. Each step in learning how to live more informed each day allows the student to develop positive reflections on their **sense and receive path struggles**. This process involves redefining their sense of self in relation to their sense of feel for self, others, and the environment, while continuously formatting **brain, body, and sense transformations** of energy, action, and feelings.

7.   Get out of your own way.

Do you **feel** for your brain? The **crisis of self** forms within the context of how you sense contact and receive interaction. Do you react without thought, or do you respond with reflection? Is your body acting in the lead of your brain, or is your brain leading your body? Which do you feel more strongly—the reactions of your body or the responses of your brain? Do you become more **mental, physical, or emotional**?**Feeling Systems Science** allows you to assess how you come to feel your brain, body, and sense systems. In the epilogue of my 2010 book, *The Information Processing Age*, we introduced the term **feeling systems theory**. You can feel my words here, but you must choose either the positive or negative path to experience the right changes within yourself—within your brain and body. To do this, you must learn how to manage the way you feel things by either accepting or resisting the flow of energy, action, and feelings through your brain, body, and sense interplay. This is a process cycle that defines how you **live, learn, think, and respond** based on how this interplay causes you to feel.

When you **sense, feel, and focus**, you bridge the connection between body and brain, linking feelings of self and mind. The **sense, feel, and focus process cycle** is a practical approach to learning how it feels when your brain leads your body. However, each step—sensing, feeling, and focusing—requires **signs of care** from your sense of feel for self, as the body undergoes neuro-physical transformation, following the brain's lead. Learning this means that the **physics of self** transitions into the **neuro-physics of the brain's body**, a core concept in **Feeling Systems Science**.

When your body reveals **signs of care**, you can actually feel these changes occurring.

Care is a goal that enables you to feel the flow of energy both forward and backward. A **sense of feel for self-care** requires respect for self, which is why understanding the body as a physical entity offers a rational perspective. The body is physical, and each time you choose to **sense and feel yourself**, the body becomes social and physical proof of your existence. Every time you respond to contact with **signs of care for yourself**, you build a stronger **sense of feel** for your **character**.

Character is a **social sign of self**, where you can observe physical proof of the brain leading the body through acts of care. This **sense of feel** allows you to focus your attention on social and environmental contact and interaction. You can feel yourself move through social contact, emerging as an environmental influence—an observable goal.**Character** transforms through the goal of learning how it feels to think and reflect on the social experience of contact. Becoming more **mental** is an outcome you want to explore, achieved through **feelings of thought** with reflection that informs and shapes your sense of self. In this **process loop**, **discipline** and **focus** arise from how you choose to sense and feel the flow of information or emotion. Living through discomfort becomes a reality-based learning experience that motivates you to care, feel, and think, helping you reflect on these actions and become more **mental**.

Progressive Investing Model 8

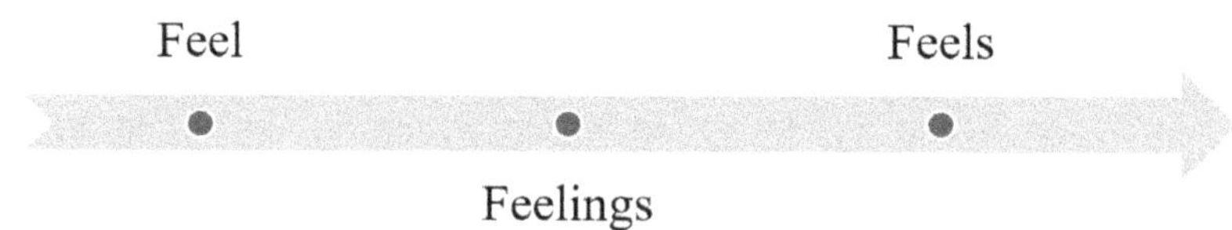

When you **feel contact** through **signs of care**, the body starts to feel like your mind. **Feelings of reflection**, influenced by the environment, shape how you respond to cooperation or participation in the **receive path functions** moving backward. For instance, when you say, *"In my mind,"* you are forming a response based on the feelings influenced by your surroundings—whether from yourself, other people, or the environment—creating a **sense of the experience**. The goal of feeling, in this case, is to observe your body's feelings long enough for that experience to transfer into thought and **bridge with reflection**, enabling you to become more mental.

You want to understand how you become more mental or reflect backward to make sense of your **self-reflection** as part of the experience. **Backward and forward feed** from self-reflection can create both good and bad feelings in your body and mind, but **forward feed** helps prepare you to manage, control, and process the ongoing experience of self. The act of feeling is also the act of sensing and focusing **feelings of care**, where the **receive path** helps connect how it feels to become more mental.

Through the way you experience contact, you receive a **sense of self**, which allows you to process how it feels to interact with your feelings of self, others, and the environment. This leads to an informed response. When you engage in **self-reflection**, you want to deepen your understanding of your **brain's body**.

In other words, you must learn how to step out of your brain's way by realizing ways to help yourself and others move through interaction. This is a **practice of self-leadership**. Learning through a **sense of feel for self** and allowing the brain to lead the body demonstrates an acceptance of **brain talk**. While we can all feel our inner voice, not everyone can transition to brain talk due to struggles with pain, hurt, sadness, anger, fear, or anxiety. The practical way to navigate through negative energy is by practicing **sense and receive path research**, which includes brain, body, and sense messaging as well as feedback loops.

Your brain is a **social organ**, living through action and learning to perform through the **mechanics of sense and receive path influences**. Consider these questions:

1. Do you **read** to your brain or your body?
2. Do you **write** to your brain or your body?
3. Do you **draw** to your brain or your body?
4. Do you **act** to your brain or your body?
5. Do you **perform** to your brain or your body?

6. Do you know how your **brain talks back**?

In each step, you are connecting the **energy of your brain** to the **actions of your body** and the **feelings of your senses** to self-learning. How you move through contact, interact, and choose to cooperate shapes your forward and backward feed, advancing your participation in the learning process.

PART TWO

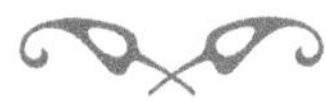

*Learn how the **brain talks back**—this is the essence of the **crisis of self**: the way you sense and receive information. To navigate this, you must be **learnable** from where you are in your thinking and responding. When you find yourself in a self-crisis, look within. Be open to learning. Don't be afraid to explore your human system. Can you apply the word **"learnable"** to yourself?*

*__Self-learning__ is a skill you must master, as it reflects signs of self-care. You should be able to feel your **inner voice** guiding you toward becoming learnable. In other words, you should feel yourself beginning to understand why you do what you do and say what you say. As you transform from your sense of self to your sense of feel for self and your brain, ask yourself: Are you **learnable?** Are these feelings reflecting **self-care?***

8.   Talk to the Brain.

People **People Who Should Review These Theories**: Those who encounter difficulties with **sense contact**, or work with individuals who struggle to interact without showing signs of anger, fear, or anxiety. Understanding how your brain talks back through your **inner voice** is key to recognizing how your sense of feel for self and your brain respond. This approach enables you to teach or observe **signs of care**.

Talking to the brain is an authentic learning strategy that involves understanding what motivates your inner voice to respond. How you choose to live, learn, and interact each day shapes the way you engage with people in your home, your environment, and your social circles. These are **progressive investing strategies** in self-learning, through intentional **brain, body, and sense activities** that influence how you think, reflect, and sense your feel for self as it leads your body.

These theories help you apply your knowledge of social interactions using special words, and they guide how you respond and cooperate with others daily.

Individuals who study **human developmental challenges** may find value in the special language we use to explore the **body-mind conflict**—concepts like the sense of self and brain-body connections, through a sense of feel for self. This approach takes into account the **social, environmental, and neural interplay**, as well as the flow of **emotion, thought, reflection**, and **forward and backward feed**.

Progressive Investing Model 9

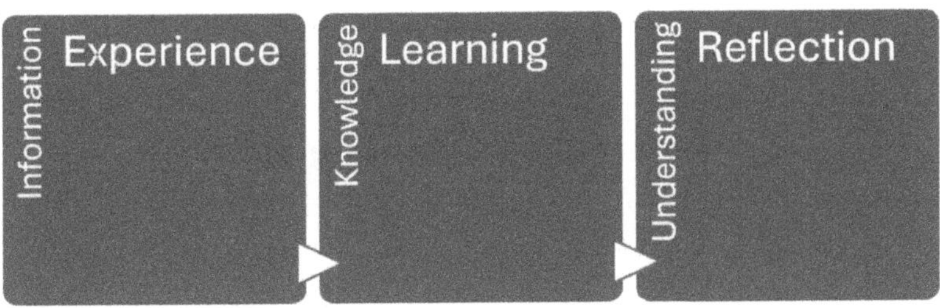

Damage to brain, body, and sense connections can manifest as **sense and receive path problems**, affecting how you process information through contact and environmental interactions. For example, when you're unable to experience contact with yourself, others, or the environment, it disrupts the **sense path**. Sense data must travel through the sense path to generate information flow into the **receive path**, where mental processing occurs.

In our studies of the human system—examining **brain, body, and sense responses** to contact and interaction—we classified **home, school, neighborhood, and workplace networks** as major life events that can influence **pain, hurt, and sadness**, damaging a person's **sense of feel for self**. This also includes the **inner voice**, as brain, body, and sense connections contribute to how we experience ourselves, others, and the environment.

As you navigate the **crisis of self**, other people, and the environment, the focus is on personal growth, academic achievement, social enrichment, and occupational skills, which serve as **experience-based self-care** strategies:

1. **Living through family decline**: You can learn how to live using **home-based learning games** to act on how contact in the home feels.

2. **Overcoming school failure**: You can learn to succeed by using **school-based learning games** to reflect on how you interact in school and how it feels to achieve success.

3. **Addressing delinquency**: You can learn by choosing to cooperate in **neighborhood vocational opportunities,** which helps foster a sense of contribution.

4. **Developing employable skills**: You can grow by choosing to participate in **distant learning options** to address skill gaps.

5. **Coping with poverty**: You can perform through **community-based learning** to improve how you engage and respond to challenges.

At each stage, you learn to leverage the resources available to you:

- Use the home you have access to.

- Use the school you attend.

- Use the neighborhood around you.

- Use the workplace where you have successful interactions.

The **crisis of self** can cause you to act as if you dislike yourself, when in reality, you are simply uncomfortable with contact or the crossover experience of another person's interaction, which makes you feel uncertain. As a result, you might not feel the need to respond. In my experience, human problems are often riddles of **sense and receive path damages**, caused by the way social contact feels or by the environments of home, school, and neighborhood networks, which spread the **pain, hurt, and sadness** of those who have experienced them as places of poor interaction. In other words, **negative experiences of contact** can lead to self-defeating behaviors that disrupt **brain, body, and sense connections**, hindering your ability to think, reflect, and manage emotions.

When you use your home to practice living through the **crisis of self**, you are focusing your **inner voice**. When you use your school to study how you interact with others through this crisis, your inner voice begins to transform the way you communicate with your brain. Each step is part of the ongoing process loop: **sensing contact, feeling interaction**, and **focusing on cooperation** to respond through **brain talk**. This means using your brain to manage energy, your body to control action, and your feelings to process how it feels to experience your social and emotional self working together. It feels empowering to be in control, with your brain leading your body.

However, if you show a **lack of care for yourself**, your sense of respect for self may lack thought and reflection, preventing you from fully understanding your experiences. When your **sense of feel** is damaged by environmental influences and you choose not to respond, your inner voice may lead you to resist contact. This resistance can block the transfer of feelings to the nervous system, making emotions less managed, controlled, or processed. In turn, this can affect how you think, respond, and release emotions moving forward.

9. Self-Research of Brain, Body, and Sense Communication.

When you study your body, you develop a **sense of self**. To truly understand how your body lives, you must also study your brain. By examining both your body and brain, **sense and receive path functions** naturally evolve as part of your **self-research**. This is why your brain takes the lead over your body, receiving information through the senses. Your brain uses your body to develop a **sense of feel for self**, which you experience every time you read, write, draw, act, or perform—expressing yourself through **brain talk**.

Progressive Investing Model 10

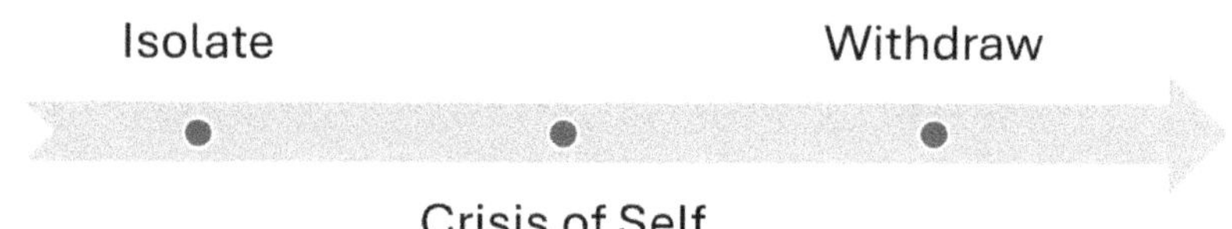

When you **isolate**, you can regress into negative states of mind. Similarly, when you **withdraw**, you can disrupt your **sense, feel, and focus process loop**. The **crisis of self** can emerge from this disconnection, affecting how you sense contact and receive neural interaction. In other words, isolating removes your **sense of feel**, and withdrawing from focus blunts the release of **signs of care**.

I am referring to **major life events** that impact **sense and receive path functions**. Feelings of hurt, pain, and sadness can lead to isolation or withdrawal from social contact, often influenced by the environment. In such cases, **therapeutic interventions** may be needed to help individuals reconnect their sense of feel, enabling the brain to act through the crisis of self. The goal of **Progressive Investing** is to practice acting through feelings of pain, hurt, and sadness, developing greater awareness by moving through the experience of self and social contact. This involves **sensing, feeling, and focusing** on sense and receive path interactions.

As you engage in **self-informing**, the receive path shifts to process how you respond to self-help. You **invest in yourself** to become more informed, through the study of **brain and body connections**.

Thus, **progressive investing** is the **action learning theory** presented throughout this book. Learning to live through the experience of self hinges on how you choose to invest in yourself daily, cultivating **self-motivation**. As you learn to motivate yourself, your **sense of feel** guides you to live each day with the aim of informing the brain, disciplining the body, and focusing the senses. You want to **feel and focus** on how it feels to experience brain, body, and sense interactions simultaneously. The **desire to learn** helps you become more aware of social and environmental processes. This includes the goal to develop the **urge to live**, navigating both negative and positive energy, or changes in states of mind, as forward-moving reflections of yourself.

Becoming more aware of your **brain leading your body** is a crucial process within the **sense path**. Your senses send signals from your body to your brain, allowing you to transition from a **sense of self** to a **sense of feel for self and the brain**, sustaining your emerging knowledge base. This is why **human systems science** is the study of brain, body, and sense systems—it enables you to explore how your brain uses your senses to structure your body's responses. From theory to practice, human systems science lets you experience your brain's workings as **backward** or **forward feed**, depending on how you interact with yourself or others. Your brain learns through your sense of feel for self, guiding your body through the **crisis of self**.

This design of human systems science is particularly beneficial for those who may suffer from **sense and receive path damage** without realizing it, as they might operate primarily through body-mind response patterns instead of learning how to navigate life through **neuro experiences**. These include the flow of information, knowledge, and understanding, all driven by a sense of feel for how the body reacts, how the brain responds, and how the senses transfer feelings. It's about learning with the **brain in the lead of the body—** understanding how to live through problems at home, learn through challenges at school, think through difficulties in the neighborhood, and respond to issues at work. Each step involves setting practical goals to guide you through the **crisis of self** in relation to others and the environment.

As you progress, you develop **thought with reflection**, which enhances your ability to sense, feel, and focus your emotions. The more you practice acting through feelings of pain, hurt, and sadness, the better you become at detecting and processing these emotions. Learning about yourself is a form of **self-research**. You come to realize that your brain must always lead your responses, using your **sense of feel for self** as a tool for self-help.

To facilitate this pivot, **human systems research** prepares you to study yourself and the events you want to move beyond in the **crisis of self**. This involves entering each situation with an awareness of how to check yourself for any signs or feelings of emotion that could cloud your judgment. A **sense of feel for self** takes the lead, respecting the challenges of contact and interaction in homes, schools, neighborhoods, and workplaces—networks not always designed to support your brain's lead over your body.

In these **fields of experience** home, school, neighborhood, and workplace networks—being prepared is essential because you feel everything in these environments. **Human Systems Research** is particularly relevant for those affected by major life events involving social contact within these settings, and the environmental influences that shape how they sense and receive information to live, learn, think, and respond to themselves, others, and the world around them. Your ability to sense and feel the transfer of emotions, both forward and backward, evolves through the capacity to become more mental, helping to reverse the negative impact on **brain-body connections** and to effect changes in yourself. The challenge is navigating contact with others who openly carry and spread their own hurt, pain, and sadness.

When you don't know how to **talk to the brain**, or when you live solely through introspection without reflecting on the things you feel, you may care less about how you transfer your **negative energy** to others. Stop! This is the **crisis of a non-reflective self**—someone who may be unwilling or unable to come to terms with their failure to show signs of care for themselves, others, and the environment.

Think of it this way: you **sense and feel for self** to remove yourself from the crisis, which then enables a clearer sense of feel for both yourself and the other person's brain to engage with. Even if they respond with signs of pain, hurt, or sadness, your **receive path** is already in **self-reflection** mode, responding to how you've chosen to act through the experience. This helps inform and discipline your brain and body connection to stay focused. In this process, both your **sense of self** and **sense of feel for self** interconnect, preparing you to perform with greater awareness.

Systems Feeling Science explores how you **feel your way** through the experience of brain, body, and sense interplay. In essence, it's the study of how you interpret and respond to contact and interaction through feelings shaped by environmental influences. These influences guide you in **comprehending brain, body, and sense process loops**. How you feel is what makes your human system a form of **technology**—when you practice acting through your experiences long enough, you generate **backward feed**. This reflection allows you to process **social contact** and **environmental influences**, advancing your **self-analysis** through feelings of **self-research**, **self-help**, and **self-discovery**.

When you choose to learn through the experience of contact, the transition to the **receive path** becomes an act of becoming more informed about how your body feels. However, if you withdraw from interaction, it impacts how your **sense of self** feels and how the brain responds. In other words, the transition to a **feeling system experience** of the receive path weakens.

This is why there's a difference between experiencing a **sense of self** through contact and transitioning to a **sense of feel for self**, where the brain leads the body. Isolating from this **sense of feel for self** and the brain weakens the proof of cooperation—your body may no longer appear under the control of the receive path. Acts like focusing on how you move through contact and interact are signs of **cooperation through physical discipline**.

10.   Dr. Slaton Live™ is the trademark for talking to the brain.

The way I express my **energy** is through **brain talk**, which reflects my **sense of feel** for parents and children in crisis. This serves as both an act of self-care and a process of self-help. Through this process, I learn how my brain processes contact and interaction, depending on how I choose to cooperate. I think and reflect on the **neuro-physics** of learning self, informed by my study of other people's contact and interaction with their environment.

As my son Chris would say, **"Speak the Truth."** This concept shapes the intellectual foundation of **human systems science** and forms the basis of **Brain Talk**. The idea of "Speak the Truth" applies in several key ways:

1) When you need to learn how to improve your ability to **live.**

2) When you need to practice **learning how to learn.**

3) When you need to write **evidence-based reports** on **sense and receive path research.**

4) When you need to assess how **children, youths, and young adults** are learning today.

5) When you need to **investigate self**, others, and their environments.

6) When you need to explore new methods to **investigate human problems,** both natural and mechanical.

7) When you need to deepen your understanding of **sense and receive path research** and the connections between **brain, body, and sense systems.**

8) When you need to **build human assets** that invest in **self-learning**, collaboration with others, and environmental learning.

9) When you need to find ways to improve the **home, school, neighborhood, and workplace networks** of children, parents, teachers, social workers, and other health professionals.

10) When you need to learn ways to **plan, organize, and implement self-care education** for stakeholders in crisis.

11) When you need to learn **Feeling Systems Science** for **mental, physical, and emotional healing** (Slaton, 2009).

Study contact in the home: When you are in crisis, you seek to understand the **physics of self-identification** because of how you experience contact within your **sense path**. It becomes essential to assess your body as you navigate struggles between **emotion, thought, and reflection**, all of which revolve around your mental awareness of self. **Self-contact** is a form of communication through how your body feels and moves in contact with others and the environment. This is the context of **human systems research**, where you practice **entering and exiting contact** in the home, learning how to move through your feelings of self in relation to others and the environment. This helps you comprehend the **physical and mental transformations** that occur through the flow of information.

Study interaction in school: Strategically, I sent my son to school to learn how to interact through his **crisis of self**. But first, he had to understand the **physics of his body**. To overcome **sense and receive path problems**, the receive path needed to be aligned with the crisis of self, experienced as part of learning. However, it was *me* who had to first comprehend the experience of learning through interaction, as part of the **neuro-physics of self-identification**. I needed to be able to read and interpret his search for self, the journey he was traversing. In **feeling systems science**, you act through feelings of hurt to learn how to navigate your body's physics, transferring acts of **self-movement** into interaction with others in the school environment.

Study cooperation in the neighborhood: This is where your child might struggle the most—making sense of **states of mind** and **feelings of thought, reflection, and emotion**. The body's language and the brain's inner voice often clash, causing confusion between **sense and receive path transactions**. Chris needed to cooperate with these experiences to understand how his **crisis of self** was evolving across three domains: contact in the home, interaction in the school, and cooperation in the neighborhood. His brain had to lead through a **sense of feel for self**, focusing on what was happening inside his body to comprehend the need for **cooperation** through signs of care. This process required thinking through feelings of self—connecting **brain, body, and sense messaging**—while using the neighborhood as a laboratory to study how people relate to **human physics** and **mentalism**.

Progressive Investing Model 11

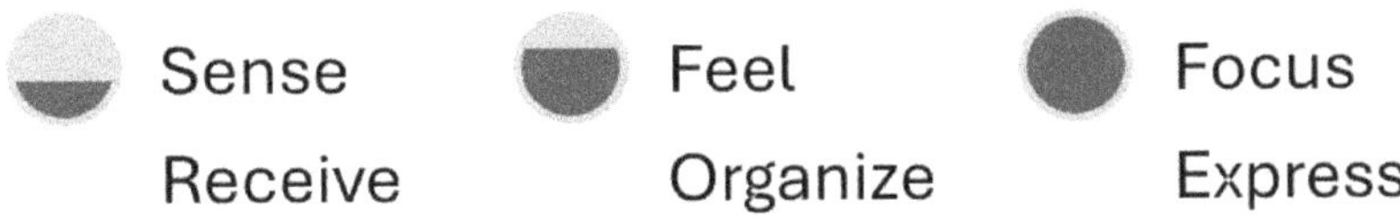

1. **Sense**: Observe the action of the body for signs of emotion. Look to define levels of control.

- ○ **Receive**: Identify behavior issues that affect the control of the brain, body, and senses.
2. **Feel**: Assess the energy of the brain for signs of thought. Measure actions that manage levels of care.
    - ○ **Organize**: Address learning problems that affect brain, body, and sense coordination.
3. **Focus**: Analyze mental feelings of the senses for signs of reflection. Symbolize processes that allow you to think through emotions.
    - ○ **Express**: Explore thinking concerns that influence brain, body, and sense messaging.

Study the workplace: This environment is best suited to evaluate communication, participation, and support processes. My son Chris chose the home as his place of self-evaluation, where he could explore the transfer from his **sense of self** to his **sense of feel for self**. He would read, write, draw, act, and perform to his brain, transitioning from his inner voice to **brain talk**. This served as proof of his participation in the process of developing **self-care** for himself, others, and the environment.

Cathartically, Chris learned to engage with his **brain's body**—growing up in crisis, which posed a threat to himself, others, and the environment—but maintaining the **character** to experience his **sense of feel for self** and keep the brain in the lead of the body.

Despite his fears, he never gave in. Instead, he consistently practiced **brain talk**, responding to feedback from his physical communication signs. Both socially and academically, Chris performed through his inner voices, developing an understanding of the **language of brain talk**. The feedback he received from how he conducted himself at home, interacted with others in school, and cooperated with family, friends, and neighbors, allowed him to act through feelings of **pain, hurt, and sadness**. Ultimately, he learned to perform as a **brain talker**.

Chris had the **courage** to express his interpretations and confront the **truth** about the crisis of self. This is **brain talk**—when you read aloud, write words, draw images that capture the experience, act to display the transformation between the **physics of the body** and the **neuro-physics of self**, and perform to integrate it all as a **sense of self**. Through this process, Chris navigated his **sense of feel for self** with the brain leading the body.

His **brain's body** described how the brain talks back through the **experience of self** in relation to other people and the environment. He worked diligently through **conduct deficits**, learning to master **brain, body, and sense communications**. Most importantly, Chris began to understand **mental health** as an ongoing effort to **inform, instruct, motivate**, and **express success** through brain talk—whether at home, in school, within his neighborhood, or in the workplace.

11. Choose the need to comprehend changes in self.

You want to learn **sense and receive path functions** as part of **self-research**, to study how you make choices and decisions. The way you **sense the affects of emotion** and **receive the effects of thought** depends on your ability to shift from a **sense of the experience** to a **sense of feel for your brain leading your body**. Your **sense of self** refers to the **physics of self**, the body-mind connection. Your **sense of feel for self** refers to the **neuro-physics** of your brain-body connections. You are the one who determines these **transformations of self**.

This is what your **brain** intends to achieve through your **sense of feel for self**—to learn how to solve **social and environmental problems** through **self-learning**. That is the purpose of **reflection**. As humans, we can choose to accept or reject experiences, allowing us to understand how to learn from changes that occur in our participation. This is why it's important to act through your **sense of self**, to learn how you perform with your **sense of feel for self** and your brain. Through this process, you think, reflect, and process emotion, becoming more aware of your sense of feel for self. This awareness helps frame the flow of information to better comprehend the **social impact** of your contact with others.

For example, **character** is reflected in physical signs of **thought, reflection, and emotion**, with the **brain leading the body**.

Progressive investing Model 12

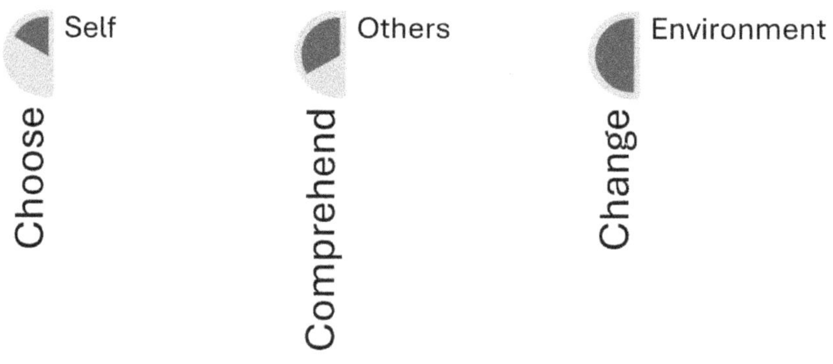

The goal is to **structure your contact with others** so that you can sense and feel the experience of **self and the brain leading the body**. This involves recognizing how you **think, reflect, and release emotion** as part of your brain's **receive path functions** in response to **social and environmental conflicts**. Your **self-character** includes the way you interact with and are influenced by your environment, where you can sense the need to change within your **body-mind** connection in order to pursue the best path toward new human learning goals. The **sense path** structures the **physics of the body**, while the **receive path** manages the **mental processes of the brain**, providing forward and backward response systems.

In other words, **emotion and thought** flow through the sense path as a result of social contact, while **thought, reflection, and emotion** arise from the receive path. This is why you must be prepared to choose the need for change to comprehend the experience of **self-knowledge**.

These elements form the foundation of how you **learn to live** through the experience of self. The **academics of self** rely on how you interpret and use your **home, school, neighborhood, and workplace networks**, which serve as foundational structures for land use and ownership worldwide. The **emotions of self** drive the spread of pain, hurt, and sadness, often resulting from **feelings of guilt, shame, and embarrassment** due to social contact and environmental influences, especially in the pursuit of rewards.

This is why you must move beyond a simple **sense of self**, where the body serves as the anchor for your **states of mind**. In this case, reflection becomes reactive—you don't need to think before reacting; instead, you generate **backward**

thought in response to the reaction. Here, you use the contact to **test the experience of self**, treating it as a **playback model** for your preferred behavior response.

On the other hand, when you move beyond a sense of self to a **sense of feel for self**, the focus shifts to the brain as the anchor, guiding your **acts to feel, think, and reflect**. This helps you balance the **effects of pain** and the **pursuit of rewards** by seeking **conscious mastery** over your brain, body, and senses. The ability to **manage, control, and focus** on self-study, while choosing to comprehend changes in your sense of self through **signs of care**, is a core human learning goal.

Just as when you **sense, feel, and focus** your brain to think through how it feels to **compete**, whether you're hurt or not, socially or environmentally, you reflect on your responses through the **neuro-physics of self**. This leads to a transformation toward higher acts of self-comprehension, ultimately helping you understand and improve your **performance**.

When you **read to the brain**, you learn not to overlook the mistakes you make. When you **write to the brain**, you acknowledge your inner voice and refuse to hide signs of care for how you feel. When you **draw to the brain**, you engage with feelings of self, others, and the environment. When you **act to the brain**, you establish your **sense of self** as the anchor for transitioning into a **sense of feel for self**, allowing the brain to lead the body. When you **perform to the brain**, you recognize how your **sense of feel** helps you choose to understand changes in **forward and backward feed**, mastering new energy impulses. You adapt to positive or negative challenges, balancing the forward and backward interplay between your **sense of self** (which reacts) and your **sense of feel** (which responds with thought and reflection).

These **feelings of self-help** enable you to manage, control, and process impulses through **sense and receive path** adjustments in emotion, thought, and reflection. These are core practices in **brain, body, and sense learning**. You come to understand the **needs of the economy** with yourself integrated into it, recognizing how your **sense of self** transfers **signs of care** through the receive path, where your inner voice guides you to feel your way through thoughts and responses.

The pressure you feel is the need to **create and appreciate process loops**—reading to inform your **sense of feel for self** and the brain, allowing you to develop products and services that address **information processing issues** in home, school, neighborhood, or workplace networks.

This is the goal of **environmental learning**. You can become an entrepreneur by using a home, school, neighborhood, or workplace network as your **learning system**. Imagine having the capacity to process **self-contact** at home, interact with others at school, and cooperate with neighborhood influences. I mean, **solving human-caused problems**. You would highlight the physical ability to move through contact to inform your **sense of self**, physically interact to discipline your **sense of feel for self**, and physically cooperate to focus on the **flow of experience, knowledge, and comprehension** of emotions, thoughts, and reflections as receive path influences of **brain talk**.

In other words, your **sense of feel for self** and your **brain in the lead of your body** is the essence of your **character**. It shapes how you think, reflect, and release emotions.

12. Self-Learning.

Realizing who you are and what you are becoming involves studying how you sense and feel to become more informed. You can see your body but not your brain, yet you instinctively know there's more to your sense of contact because you can perceive how it feels to interact. As your awareness grows, your **sense of self** transforms your **inner voice's** experience. Your **sense of feel for self** operates as a **receive path process loop**, enabling you to remain **learnable**.

Self-learning is the internal capacity to gain insights from your **contact-to-interaction** experiences. I view your **sense of self** as the **external sense path**, while your **sense of feel for self** and your brain serve as the internal transformation mechanisms through **receive path functions**. Contact brings its own influences, while interaction drives counter-influences that shape who you are and what you're becoming through how you process **information flow**. To fully understand this flow, it's essential to grasp the interplay between **sense and receive paths**—the **social physics of the body** and the **neuro-physics of the brain**—as part of **self-learning process loops**.

We all encounter **pain, hurt, and sadness**. This approach seeks to structure the experience of self and brain, recognizing that without a solid knowledge base to understand the **good and bad choices** we make, we risk missing the deeper implications of our behaviors. You can be **ugly on the outside**, as your **sense of self**, influenced by physical, social, and environmental factors, can foster negative behaviors that disrupt brain, body, and sense messaging. Alternatively, you can be **ugly on the inside** without realizing it, by avoiding the confrontation of external feelings while undergoing the transformation into the **brain's body**.

Progressive Investing Model 13

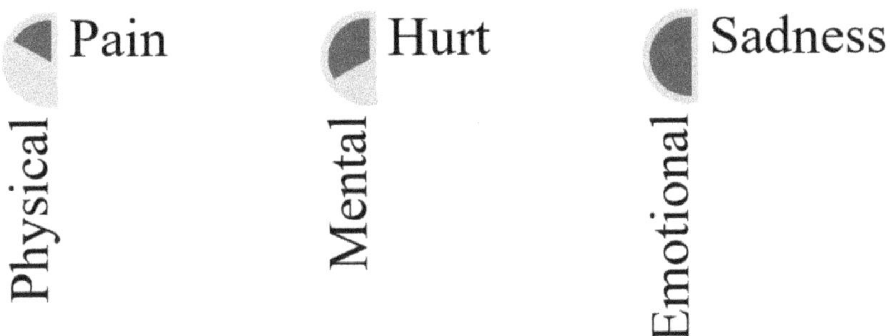

Physical pain can block the transformation of your **sense of self**. **Mental hurt** can disrupt your **sense of feel for self**. **Emotional sadness** can take a toll on how you experience both. These experiences affect the way you encounter **contact**, **neural interaction**, and **cooperation**. This is the purpose of the **Brain's Body Learning System**. Through **Dr. Slaton Live™**, you are introduced to **process learning**, using **sense and receive path research** to ground the practice of **self-learning** in relation to others and the environment. This sets the stage for integrating traditional approaches to human problem-solving with **Progressive Investing**, a method that supports **physical, mental, and emotional healing** for those not set up for traditional learning.

Learning with **Dr. Slaton Live™** involves studying **human systems science**—the interplay of **brain, body, and sense events**—to create process cycles for **self-care** and the **neuro-physics of self**. The **neuro-physics of self** refers to the **receive path** as a function of the brain, where energy flows through the self, transforming the body's actions and the feelings of the senses in response. **Dr. Slaton Live™** focuses on the study of self as **human systems research**, connecting the **process loop** of brain, body, and sense events to signs of care for others and the environment. This practice helps you learn to **live for more than just self** through the practice of **progressive investing**.

In other words, **sense and receive path learning** develops **self-awareness**, helping you navigate **pain, hurt, and sadness** each day. This awareness leads to **informing the brain, disciplining the body**, and **focusing the senses**.

The transformation of the **sense path** involves understanding how **information moves** between the body and sense receptors, seeking connections between the brain and body to establish **receive path functions**. These functions transfer **sense data** through a **sense of feel for self**, with the brain establishing ways to interpret the body's experiences, ensuring that a **feedback loop** allows you to comprehend your responses. **Acts of self-care** enable you to sense, feel, and focus on the forward and backward flows of **energy, action, and feelings** as you become more aware. As the brain takes the lead, it organizes **emotion, thought, and reflection**, unfolding the **synthesis** of these experiences and deepening the **analysis of self-participation**.

You **receive** in order to **accept a sense of feel**. You process **brain and body connections** to experience the environment through your senses, interpreting feelings. You respond to **brain, body, and sense messaging** as part of **sense and receive path research**, which allows you to receive, organize, and express feedback. This feedback helps you understand how you live through **physical feelings of pain**, learn through **mental feelings of hurt**, and think through **emotional feelings of sadness**—all as **neuro-physical signs of self-care**. These signs represent how you care for yourself, others, and the environment. Through **Dr. Slaton Live™**,

human systems science explains how a **brain, body, and sense messaging knowledge base** is built using special words that connect with the human experience of **living in a home, learning in a school, thinking in a neighborhood**, and **responding in a workplace**.

The **knowledge base** for solving **sense and receive path problems** is designed for individuals who have been affected by major life events within their **home, school, neighborhood, and workplace networks**. This platform serves as a foundation for **self-learning**. In essence, this is **self-science**, aimed at improving how people learn to navigate **social contact** and **environmental influences**. It helps individuals cope with **pain, hurt, and sadness** by transitioning from a **sense of self** to a **sense of feel for self**. You learn how to respond to the experiences of **brain, body, and sense messaging** as **neural influences**.

This process structures ways to live through a **sense of self-contact**, and interact with the goal of learning how to accept a **sense of feel for self** and the brain, as they influence your senses. Your **knowledge base** is self-engineered through **cooperative forward and backward feedback loops**, which sustain **sense and receive path research**.

13.   Self-Reflective Research.

Memory is formed through the experience of **sense contact** and the influential ways you interact. I refer to this as a **mind state**, a **self-reflective state** of reacting or responding. You learn to distinguish between **past and present emotions**, **thoughts**, and **reflections** by studying how you sense contact and feel **neural interaction**. When the brain leads the body in responding, you experience **forward feed**.

Self-reflective research unpacks what happens between your **sense of self** and your **sense of feel for self**. Learning about yourself within the framework of **brain learning** builds upon **sense and receive path research**, forming a **process loop** of self-reflective practices. The relationship between the self, the brain, the body, and the senses is crucial in understanding both the **physics of self** and the **neuro-physical transformations** of self. Self-reflective research operates under the assumption that the brain is in the lead of the body, with **sense contact** serving as proof of self-performance through a **sense of feel** for what occurred.

The goal of reflection is to **comprehend self-action** and how you respond to yourself, others, and the environment. In **human systems science**, when you sense, you feel; when you feel, you receive; when you receive, you process; and when you process, you focus the **neuro-physics of self** with the brain leading the body. In other words, you manage **sense contact** and **environmental interaction** to control the flow of feelings as **neural feedback**, enabling focused responses to experiences.

The confluence of **emotion, thought,** and **reflection**—as the synthesis of sense and receive path processing—creates the capacity for **self-reflective research**. By focusing on your emotions, you can feel your thoughts. When you focus and feel both emotions and thoughts moving through your **sense and receive path interplay**, you experience **reflection** as both **backward and forward feed**.

Progressive Investing Perspective Model 14

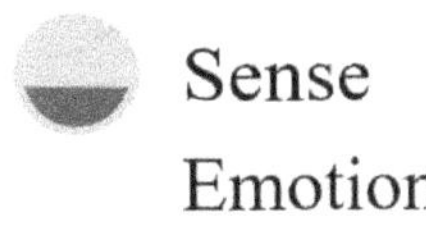 Sense
Emotion

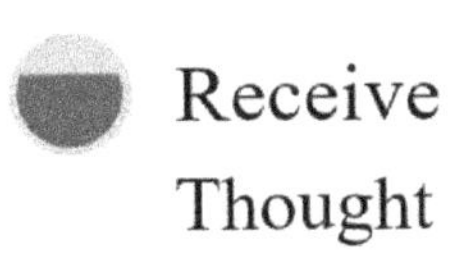 Receive
Thought

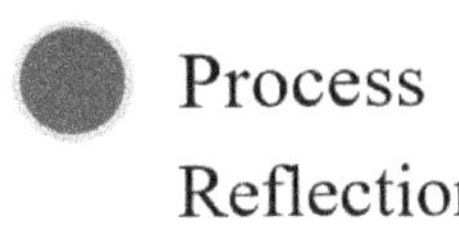 Process
Reflection

When you live with a **damaged sense path**, it's crucial to learn how this affects your **receive path**. A **sense of feel for self** draws on the **brain and body connections**, helping you understand how you sense contact and receive interaction as **social and environmental influences** on your neural processes. The ability to move through contact enhances your capacity to reflect on experiences and recognize these process variables as part of your **sense and receive path functions**. When you reflect on your sense of feel for self, you engage in **sense and receive path research**, which heightens your awareness of the roles played by **emotion, thought**, and **reflection** in **forward and backward feed process loops**.

Since 1982, I have continuously studied **education and science**, seeking answers to issues such as **family decline, school failure, delinquency, lack of employable skills**, and **poverty**—all of which have shaped my evolving concepts of **self-learning**. As a **human learning consultant**, I've applied these studies to critique, appraise, and evaluate how individuals struggling with **living, learning, thinking**, and **responding** in their **home, school, neighborhood, and workplace networks** respond to contact and environmental interaction. My research includes studying parents and children in crisis due to these major life events, objectively reviewing how they **receive information** and respond to **discipline**.

This includes **social and emotional learning** for children, youths, young adults, and adults, as well as **social and**

economic learning for parents who struggle with reading, writing, drawing, acting, and performing with their **brain in the lead of the body**. This problem becomes more complex when individuals have not been prepared for the experience of **contact** or the mechanics of **interaction** that train them to think without a sense of feel for self and the brain. It's more challenging to connect how you feel contact with reflection when you haven't learned to accept how contact feels and how your brain responds to it. These are the **acts of self-research**, explored through the lens of **self-reflective research**.

In 2021, the COVID-19 pandemic forced me to close my offices. Simultaneously, my wife endured a stroke, prompting me to take a sabbatical and adjust my practice. My wife, who had served as my research assistant since 1995, became the focus of my study on how people with **damaged sense and receive path functions** receive information and respond to environmental interaction. Implementing a **self-research approach**, we began working together to understand her experience of **memory loss**, further highlighting the importance of studying self in relation to others. Her experience of contact became mine, and my experience of interaction became her responses to my **brain talk**.

This set a new foundation for **human systems science**, broadening the study of the **neuro-physics of self**: the brain leading the body through an emergent cycle of **sense, feel, and focus**. The practice of **self-learning** focuses on recognizing **contact** as a sense of self and **interaction** as a sense of feel for that interplay, observing how the neuro-physics of self responds through signs of care. The goal is to engage the **sense path** as the driving force to feel and focus on signs of care, acknowledging that the interaction may provoke mental confusion or anger, particularly when influenced by feelings of **memory loss**. This is why **care** plays a central role throughout my **education and science literature**. My wife, **Dr. Dolores Slaton**, is a key figure whose **voice and experience** runs through this book as **brain talk**. All **brain talk** is grounded in **sense and receive path research**, and I express this as the privilege of experiencing education and science repeatedly—through the study of **self**, **other people**, and the **environment**. This stems from long-standing, participant-driven research bonds. In essence, learning how we inform the brain, discipline the body, and focus the senses in response to experiences of self, others, and the environment involves the active assessment of **mental activity** and **self-talk**. As we navigate the challenges of **mindfulness** and **forgetfulness**, we review our responses to one another's contact and interaction, engaging in dialogue about **sense and receive path experiences** from multiple perspectives through **brain talk**. In this process, the brain takes the lead, guiding the body to **self-actualize**, inform, and discipline the senses in response to contact and environmental interactions.

This approach has helped Dolores move forward, particularly through her **recollections** of fieldwork with parents and children in crisis who face similar **sense and receive path problems**. Our day-to-day dialogues have made the concept of **forward and backward feed** clearer. For instance, each morning, Dolores makes it a point to join me in my study lab, where I ask her, "What's going on? How are you feeling? Is anything on your mind?" Gradually, this practice has helped her to **sense and feel** her way to respond, allowing us to assess her progress. Dolores actively participates in this writing process by reflecting on her experiences, clarifying language, and confirming her understanding in relation to **self-research**. This assures me that she is working to make sense of my work and is engaged in her own recovery.

14. The Brain's Body.

The way you sense and receive the flow of **energy**, **action**, and **feelings** is at the core of how you navigate through the affects of **emotions** and the effects of **thought**. To manage this flow effectively, you must engage with the processes that inform your **brain**, discipline your **body**, and process your **senses** as **neuro influences** that bridge your brain-body connection. A **sense of feel for self** and the **brain in the lead of the body** means being aware of and responding to changes in body language, states of mind, and behaviors. These changes reflect the **receive path** process loops that move you forward.

The **brain's body** is a term that describes how you engage with sense and receive path performance. It's about transforming your **sense of self** into a **sense of feel for self**, with the brain leading the body. Managing this flow of information is critical for building **knowledge**, allowing you to understand and respond to changes within yourself. Rather than isolating to resist contact or withdrawing to reject interaction, you engage in a process of searching for your **character** through receive path transformations. This involves actively choosing to **think**, **reflect**, and release **managed emotions** to respond to life's challenges.

When you consciously process your sense of self, you can feel the **chemical** and **biological exchanges** taking place within you as proof of transformation. These sensations help you understand that the **brain must act in the lead of the body**, guiding you through the **sense, feel, and focus** process loop that enables the flow of energy, action, and feelings, ultimately shaping **memory** and **recall**.

For those who have been hurt by major life events, it can be difficult to pinpoint the experiences that trigger the flow of **anger**, which can lead to a fear of contact and interaction. This fear often manifests as anxiety and a resistance to processing your sense of self. Your sense of self is how you interpret the **mental physics** of the body as you move through social contact, requiring you to interact through feelings of thought that are connected to **brain-body transitions** and **reflective research**. These transitions are crucial, as they allow you to process how you **look**, **act**, and **feel** about the experiences that shape your mental growth.

Failing to make these brain-body transitions leads to a disconnection from your ability to **sense**, **feel**, and **focus** on the mental and physical aspects of managing emotions. Without this connection, the crisis of self becomes harder to navigate, leaving you more vulnerable to being emotionally overwhelmed rather than empowered to respond constructively. The ability to embrace being upset as a necessary part of growth—rather than something to avoid— gives you the power to manage and control the crisis of self.

Progressive Investing Model 15

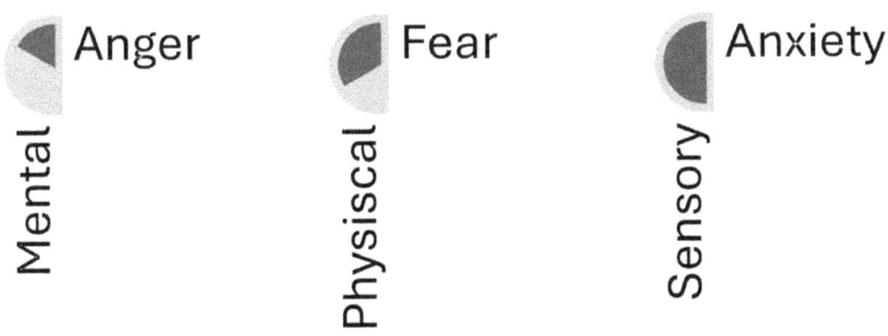

Becoming aware of the neuro physics of self involves understanding how your **mental**, **physical**, and **sensory**

organization connect your **brain**, **body**, and **senses**. This is what I call the neuro physics of self—a study that brings into focus how these systems work together. By learning to detect what has happened to you, how it happened, and where it happened, you gain the tools to perform **self-analysis**. This reflective practice allows you to answer the deeper question: **Why** is this happening to you? When you begin to comprehend the brain's body, it enhances your **critical thinking skills**, helping you navigate the **crisis of self**—how you live, how you learn, how you think, and how you respond to social and environmental contact.

As you convalesce from a **lack of self-care** and focus, the key question to ask is: **Why is your brain your body?** Inside your body, a vast network of **nerve tissue** is connected to your brain through **sense cells**, which are the messengers between brain and body. In my book *Education and Science: The Brain's Body* (2022), I describe how **brain, body, and sense organs communicate** through the nervous system. Similarly, in *Brain Talk: Learning the Brain's Body with Dr. Slaton Live™* (2024), I explore how **brain talk** happens through **sense and receive path activity**, showing how the brain continually "talks back" in a feedback loop with the body. The more you engage with your brain and think of it as **leading your body**, the more you build the capacity to navigate your thoughts, emotions, and reactions.

This understanding is crucial for **brain-body connectivity**. When you begin to **confirm a sense of feel for self**, you establish **proof of capacity**—the neuro physics of your brain leading your body. Through **sense and receive path research**, you inform yourself through signs of awareness, learning how to **discipline the body** and respond to social and environmental influences. Developing this sense of feel for self helps you recognize how to **thrive** through life's challenges. This includes learning to respond to the **affects of emotion**, **thought patterns** from others, and poor mental states.

Every day, we need to **live to learn** how to navigate these brain-body feedback loops to **inform**, **discipline**, and **process** our experiences. The more you engage with these practices, the more effectively you will think through how your **brain's body performs** and how it reflects **signs of care** in your interactions with others. Understanding these connections helps you build **self-awareness**, leading to more constructive responses to life's challenges.

Learning the brain's body with Dr. Slaton Live™ is about *talking to the brain, not the body.* This method teaches you how to enhance your awareness of the **brain, body, and senses**, focusing on how **sense and receptor cells** run from your upper to lower torso as **neurotransmitters**. As you engage with this concept, imagine how **learning the brain's body** as a human technology and practicing **brain talk** helps you understand the brain's response to **social and emotional influences**.

When you look at the images of the brain's body and the **neurotransmitters of the nervous system**, you can begin to feel the interaction between these elements. Similarly, as you read this book, you are *reading to the brain*, and the brain talks back through a process cycle of **forward and backward feed**. This process loop helps you recognize your **sense of feel for self**, creating a connection between **social contact** and **environmental interaction**.

In this cycle, your **brain is the receive path**, processing neural activity, while your **body is the sense path**, which you aim to control to navigate contact and interaction effectively. This dynamic represents the foundation of **social and emotional learning**—understanding how you **sense contact** and **transfer environmental interaction** into **neural activity** that drives your responses.

To **comprehend this process loop** of brain and body, you must develop an **unobstructed vision of self**, meaning that you must actively engage in recognizing and accepting **signs of care** for your brain and body connections. However, this can feel uncomfortable because it requires focus and awareness of how contact feels and how to focus effectively. When you can sense and feel the contact through **controlled focus**, you begin to receive contact more consciously, gaining an internal sense of how to manage your **brain, body, and sense connections**.

The **receive path process loop**—the interaction between your sense of feel for self and the brain—changes how you move through experiences. Your sense of feel is the **key** that allows you to **transfer social contact into environmental interaction** with the brain leading your body. In other words, your **sense of feel** is the process loop that enables your brain to lead the body through experiences, ensuring **states of mind** are expressed thoughtfully.

Accepting **acts of care** is crucial for comprehending how to manage and adjust your reactions. When you **look within** and focus on your **sense of feel for self**, you express **feelings of care**, which can change the way you sense, feel, and focus on brain, body, and sense messaging. If you follow the **physics of self** in relation to other people and the environment, you gain the ability to manage difficult emotions—such as **anger, fear, or anxiety**—by calming down and focusing your brain and body connections.

Once you experience a **managed self**, you gain control over your **thoughts**. This leads to a state where **thought is controlled** and **reflection and emotion** are focused in **forward feed**, resulting in an increased sense of awareness and self-care.

PART THREE

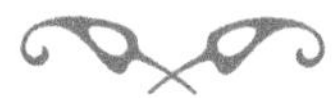

You possess an innate drive to **change the world**, fueled by a commitment to **self-learning**. Through the study of **sense and receive path research**, you assess how you experience **contact** and use this understanding to interact meaningfully with the world around you. This approach allows you to comprehend how you live through various forms of contact and informs your evolving **sense of self**. By learning to recognize how you **sense, feel, and focus your brain**, you become more attuned to shifts in your **body mind states**—allowing you to adjust, understand, and navigate your interactions with greater clarity.

The key lies in understanding how your brain and body **interact to receive, organize, and express** internal and external influences. As you master these transformations, you move toward a deeper analysis of how you cooperate through **signs of care for self** and your brain. This **synthesis of self-awareness** allows you to evaluate how you receive, process, and respond to stimuli, leading to greater control over your actions and reactions. By doing so, you enhance your ability to make conscious choices that align with your drive for personal growth and change.

15. Sense and receive path Research.

When you're in a **crisis**, physical contact alone may not be enough to establish strong **brain-body connections**. To truly understand how you sense and interact with the world, you need to study your **sense path** as a form of **physical action learning** and the **receive path** as a more subtle, often **unobservable process**. This study allows you to grasp the deeper mechanics of the **human physics of self**, focusing on how contact between yourself and others creates a **back-and-forth dialogue**—or colloquy—between your internal and external environments.

Through **sense and receive path research**, you come to realize that:

- **The brain is the body**—a unified system where physical experiences and internal processing converge.

- **Forward feed** refers to the **neural responses** that arise from interactions, while **backward feed** involves the **social cognitive flow**, where the brain reflects on these experiences and guides the body's actions.

Your **sense path** represents the body in its external form, as it navigates physical and social environments. Meanwhile, your **receive path** represents the brain's internal environment, where processing, reflection, and emotion take place.

The goal of **sense and receive path research** is to bridge the gap between the physical experiences of the body and the **neuro-physics** of the brain. This connection fosters an improved understanding of how **brain, body, and sense**

messaging work together to guide your thoughts, actions, and emotional responses, helping you move through crises with greater clarity and resilience.

Progressive Investing Model 16

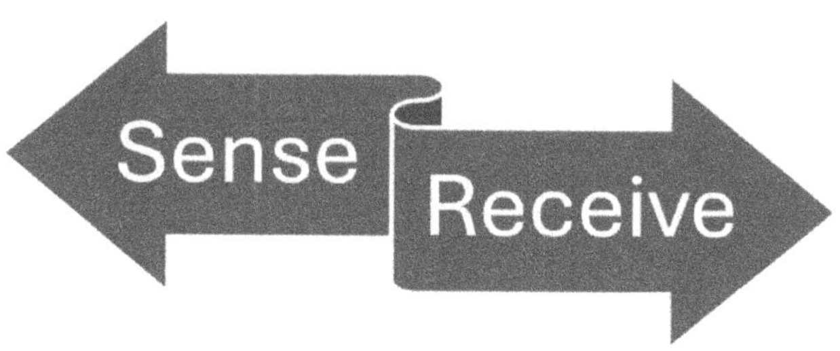

You describe the **social physics of self** as the **sense path** and the **receive path** as transformative stages leading to the **neuro-physics of self**. These stages guide **self-research**, which generates levels of **awareness** through the study of **signs of care**. This awareness encourages participation through a **sense of feel for self**, with the brain acting in the lead of the body, maintaining continuity with the social physics of self.

When you experience **hurt**, you may distance yourself from what's happening around you as a defense mechanism to avoid reliving past pain. This can lead to **sadness**, which in turn creates a lack of care in responding to yourself, leaving you seeking the information and knowledge needed for understanding. The presence of hurt and sadness may transform how you make **contact** with yourself, others, and the environment, potentially triggering **anxiety** between your **sense of self** and your **sense of feel for self**. These emotions can manifest as a reluctance to engage in **sense and receive path research**, which involves:

1. **Self-care,**
2. **Self-help,**
3. **Self-discovery**.

When you **block your sense path**, you hinder your ability to make sense of who you are in a **social context**. This block can also affect your **receive path**, preventing you from processing experiences fully. **Hurt, pain, or sadness** can limit your willingness to engage with feelings, affecting how you reflect on yourself and others. The **sense path** gathers **sense data**—information about your experiences—and if you resist acknowledging these experiences, you limit your ability to transfer them into **self-knowledge** and **understanding**. This creates a barrier to analyzing **how and why you are the way you are**.

Understanding your **participation** in life through feelings of hurt, pain, and sadness often depends on your ability to maintain a **sense of feel for self**. This **synthesis of receive path functions** often relies on a search for **signs of care**, which helps guide your **self-awareness** and encourages **healing**.

It is within your **sense of feel for self** that you find the desire to **live through crisis**, searching for **signs of care**—whether from yourself, others, or the environment. This process reflects the journey of **learning to navigate your brain's body**. The senses are designed to inform the brain via the **receive path**, and your **sense of feel for self-care** becomes a key driver in learning how to process and think through **feelings of sadness, pain, or hurt**. The way you learn to **sense, feel,** and **focus** on the **connections between self, others, and the environment** allows you to logically approach and study the **crisis of self**.

When you can act through a **sense of feel for self**, with the **brain in the lead of your body**, these are some of the greatest **signs of care** you can manifest. The process of **informing the brain**, **disciplining the body**, and **processing the senses** amalgamates your sense of feel as key technologies for **self-research**, **self-help**, and **self-discovery**. Through this, you are actively **defining what you are becoming** as you engage in **sense and receive path research**, which frees the flow of **information, experiences, knowledge**, and **understanding**. This process is crucial for managing how pain can fester and manifest as **physical resistance** to contact.

Physical signs of care can transform how you navigate your **social sense of self** to your **neural sense of feel for self**. As you encounter **sense and receive path challenges**, which test your emotional and cognitive stability, reflection from **stored states of mind**—or past experiences—often influences how you behave physically. Meanwhile, **reflection from your sense of feel for self** connects these **feelings of thought** to the way you respond to challenges along the **sense and receive path**.

If you are able to **move through feelings of hurt** and engage in **social contact**, you increase your chances of recognizing **signs of care** in your interactions. This, in turn, helps you transition more smoothly to **receive path functions**, where you can become more aware of the interplay between your **brain, body**, and **senses**. This awareness is essential for progressing through difficult experiences and moving toward greater **self-understanding** and **healing**.

Knowingly accepting the **pain**, **hurt**, or **sadness** you feel long enough to experience a shift—from **environmental influences** to **neural receive path functions**—is a powerful moment in the process of **self-care**. It allows you to **sense**, **feel**, and **focus** your energy, actions, and emotions as **signs of care**, which act as the game changer when moving through **upset sense and receive path functions** caused by major life events. Whether the disruption stems from **manmade environments**, **natural world events**, or **organic injuries**, the **crisis of self-learning** becomes much more difficult without integrating **signs of care** into the experience of social or environmental interaction. These signs help transform mental activity into constructive progress.

The **objective signs of care**—awareness of the **sense path**—and the **subjective feelings of care** for the **receive path**—forge the **process cycles** essential for moving forward. This cycle consists of:

1. **Sense, feel, focus**

2. **Receive, organize, express**

3. **Receive, process, respond through feelings of self, brain, and body.**

These **sensory**, **mental**, and **physical transitions**—from sense and receive paths—connect you to the **brain's body** and the **neuro physics of self**. As contact moves through the **sense path**, interaction transitions to the **receive path**, and the cooperation between sense and receive paths merges **brain-body connections**. Participation in this process allows you to form a **sense of feel for self**, with the **brain leading the body**. As you perform these sense and receive path tasks, you **actualize the goal** of strengthening your **brain's body**, enabling greater resilience and a deeper understanding of your personal development.

This dynamic interplay is the key to **self-learning**, helping you transform crises into opportunities for growth by maintaining focus on how your **brain**, **body**, and **senses** interact and adapt through **signs of care**.

16.   Brain Talk.

The way you **sense and feel contact** indeed activates your **inner voice**, shaping the way you experience **self-talk**. However, this can become problematic when you're not fully aware of how **self-talk** evolves in response to your **neuro energy**, **actions**, and **feelings**. For this evolution to take place effectively, your **brain** needs to be ready to receive the flow of information, your **body** must be under the control of your **sense of feel for self**, and your **senses** must focus on the exchanges of **physical** and **neuro energy**. Without this alignment, you might fall into pure **introspection**, missing out on opportunities to **participate in the informed release of responses** by leveraging the **human physics** of **brain**, **body**, and **sense messaging**.

When you first encounter contact, your **inner voice** takes hold of that experience, shaping your initial reaction. The **state of mind** in that moment influences whether you resist or accept the **self-talk** formations. This is why learning how to **feel your way through** the experience of self is critical. The **sense of feel** is where **information processing** moves to the next level, where **emotion** and **thought** may collide. This requires **focus**—allowing both your **self** and **brain** to interact through the experience of the **body**.

As the flow of your **inner voice** transitions into levels of **self-awareness**, the search for understanding why you respond the way you do emerges as **thought**, manifesting in a **reflective state**. This is where **brain talk** begins to form, as the **brain** prepares the **body** and **senses** to respond. The **examples** provided throughout this book demonstrate how this process unfolds. For instance:

- When you **write about an experience,** you are essentially **reading to the brain,** engaging its deeper processing mechanisms.

- When you **read to the brain,** you can feel the **forward** and **backward flow** of your **sense of feel for self.**

- When you **draw images** based on your **states of mind**, you engage in reflection through your **sense of feel** for self, other people, and the environment.

Similarly, when you **talk to yourself aloud**, you are engaging in **brain talk**. This is the **dialogue** between your **brain** and **body**, a conversation driven by the **flow of neural energy**, whether it's **negative** or **positive**. You may experience this flow **backward** through your **inner voice** or **forward** as introspection transforms into objective **signs** of brain, body, and sense acts. These **acts of communication** help you navigate the complexities of **self-reflection**, turning abstract emotional experiences into informed responses.

The transformation of **introspection** into **brain talk** is essential for fostering **self-awareness** and understanding the dynamics between your **sense of self** and your **sense of feel for self**.

Your **sense of self** as the **body mind** relates directly to the way you navigate **social contact** and **environmental influences**. These forces structure the **flow of energy, action,** and **feelings** that must pass through the **human system**. This is why I focus on **talking to the brain**, not the body—because it sets up the **sense and receive path interplay**. Through **signs of care**, this interplay helps to manage the effects of **emotion**, which ultimately stimulates **brain talk**.

For example, if I aim to **inform**, **discipline**, or **focus** the exchange of feelings, I seek to do so through a balanced interaction between my **sense of self** and my **sense of feel for others and the environment**. This helps to **elevate signs of care**, allowing both parties to adjust and adapt to the experience of me as I lead with my brain in control of my body.

When you act with a sense of **leading**, it flows from **self-talk** that has evolved through **brain** and **body awareness**. This awareness allows you to respond reflectively to the experience and guide your actions through **thoughts**. Therefore, your **sense of feel for self** and the brain manifests as your **inner voice**— the conduit through which **self-talk** directs the **backward flow of energy**, **action**, and **feelings** in reflective ways. This process helps interpret the **brain**, **body**, and **sense messages**.

Talking to the **brain** instead of the **body** recognizes that the **receiver of your brain talk** might be in a **state of mind** that resists your contact, potentially feeling threatened by your presence or actions. The **body** can often reflect **physical interpretations** of the **mind's behaviors**, manifesting as **pain**, **hurt**, or **sadness**—what you describe as the **body mind effect**. These physical signs can serve as cues for understanding the mental or emotional states driving these behaviors.

By focusing on **brain talk**, you're able to respect this reality and lead through the **inner voice**, using signs of care to avoid further triggering negative responses. This approach allows for more meaningful connections, helping others adjust to the experience of your interaction while you guide your **brain**, **body**, and **sense system** with intentional, reflective awareness.

Progressive Investing Model 17

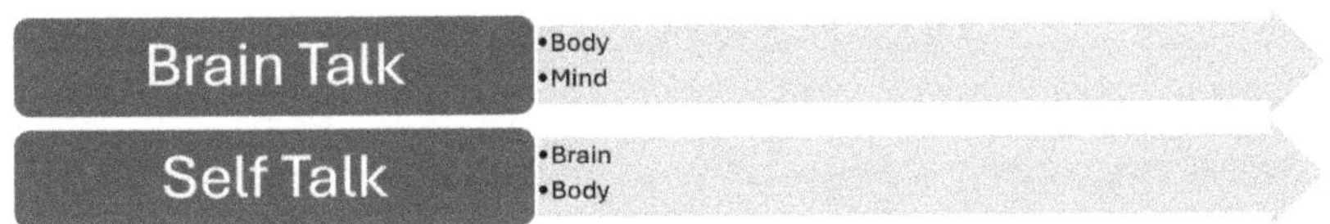

Positive **sense and receive path research** begins with **self-talk**, where you consciously choose to guide the flow of **positive energy, action**, and **feelings**. This involves becoming more aware of how you respond to both **thought** and **emotion**. By caring to listen to your **inner voice**, your **sense of feel for self** activates emotional and cognitive processes that link **sense and receive path functions** to the **brain, body**, and **sense interplay**.

Brain talk includes the exchange of **social contact** and **neural interaction**, grounded in a **sense of feel for self**, others, and the environment. This interaction helps you assess **signs of care**, providing proof that you can care for yourself, others, and the environment simultaneously—a key element of what it means to be human.

Being human is a combination of **mental, physical**, and **sensory experiences**, all driven by the flow of **energy, action**, and **feelings**. If you care about how you feel things, you naturally want to comprehend those feelings. **Care** is closely connected to how you engage in acts of living, learning, thinking, and responding to **social contact** and **environmental influences**. These factors shape your **moods** and **states of mind**. To live through the emotional impact of these experiences, you must choose to learn how to **adjust to emerging behaviors** that arise from how you sense and feel contact, especially when negative responses need to be managed and controlled as part of your **feelings of self**.

Brain talk is about reflecting on your experiences and understanding that within the **sense and receive path exchanges** lies the flow of **brain**, **body**, and **sense messaging**. These are impulses to respond and shape your awareness. **Empowering your sense of feel for self** requires care. Care, in this sense, is about learning how to manage the flow of **energy**, **action**, and **feelings** while also controlling how your brain and body respond to these influences. It involves the discipline to **focus on brain, body, and sense coaction**, which integrates **self-talk** as a powerful tool for expressing care.

You can sense the movement of **negative** or **positive energy** through your responses, which are formed from **emotion**, **thought**, and **reflection**. Acknowledging your **sense of feel** means recognizing the importance of caring enough to participate in actions that manage the flow of information. This, in turn, helps control how your body reacts to what your **senses process**. Coming to terms with your **feelings**—and the ability to experience multiple feelings at once—allows you to structure your **mental**, **physical**, and **sensory experiences**. You begin to understand how **energy**, **action**, and **feelings** impact your sense of self and influence your interactions with others and your environment.

When you train yourself not to care about how **contact feels**, you disrupt the natural flow of energy between your **sense and receive path functions**. This leads to **self-influenced challenges** within your **sense, feel, and focus cycle**, which is essential for processing and responding to the world around you. The **process loop**—the flow of receiving, processing, and responding—becomes blocked when you suppress or ignore the importance of how contact feels.

In such moments, the **preferred signs of care**, such as self-awareness and **self-help**, encounter resistance. Negative feelings, whether they stem from rejection, avoidance, or internal conflict, begin to push back against the natural flow of information. You might feel this in your **inner voice**, where you sense an internal resistance or an urge to block out the necessary adjustments needed for positive growth.

This resistance is what I refer to as the **body-mind conflict**. In this state, the **images of the body** reflect on **behavioral responses** as **states of mind** that become fixed, maintaining their own **physics of resistance to change**. These fixed states represent your reluctance to adjust, grow, or embrace transformation, and they manifest in your body's responses—whether through stress, tension, or emotional shutdowns.

On the other hand, when you align your **sense of feel for self** with active participation in the **practice of self-awareness**, you can learn to appear **cool, calm, and collected**. Your **inner voice** becomes a tool for introspection, which, when directed positively, transforms into **measurable environmental responses**. This evolution of learning helps build **intelligence** as you consciously engage in the flow of **sense and receive path functions**.

By choosing to care, you begin to guide your **inner voice** through these **decisive acts** of participating in **self-learning**. You can focus on aligning your emotions and thoughts with positive responses, allowing you to overcome the **body-mind conflict** and sustain healthier, more integrated **brain-body connections**. This care allows you to embrace change and move beyond the **resistance to growth** that hinders your ability to manage and control your responses to life's challenges.

17.   Self, Brain, Body Connections.

When you **sense contact**, the ultimate goal is to **feel your way through the experience**, using acts of **focus** to guide yourself. The **brain interacts with the body** through a **process loop** that involves both your **sense of self** and your **sense of feel for self**, with the brain in the lead. The emotional baggage—moods and mind states—can create **negative forward feed** when left unchecked, which can result in reactions. However, by recognizing and utilizing **backward feed** from the **receive path**, you engage with **signs of care** that allow you to pause, reflect, and manage your emotions. In this way, the brain leads the body through a **balanced response**.

The question of self-awareness comes into play when you ask, **What does it mean to be you?** Is it about how you define yourself, or how others define you? Is it a matter of **competition**, or is it about deeply understanding your own **brain-body connections**? These connections reveal that you are both **physical on the outside** and **neuro physical on the inside**, creating a complex system that navigates the world.

The challenge lies in how long it takes to connect the **external self**—how you appear to others—with the **internal self**, which shapes how you **respond** to yourself, other people, and the environment. This competitive struggle between others' perceptions and your own **feelings of self** is a daily conflict. You can feel these **brain and body influences** through the **senses**, and understanding these influences is key to developing self-awareness.

How long does it take to fully realize your **sense of feel for self**? This awareness comes when you allow your **brain to lead your body**, giving yourself enough time to reflect and gain value from these experiences as **self-intellect**. This concept is rooted in **Human Physics**, where the **experience of self** is studied as the **brain and body connection** that shapes how you sense and receive information.

By **observing self** and **the brain** through physical and emotional experiences, you begin to understand the dynamic interplay between your **brain and body**. The act of studying self in relation to your physical, social, emotional, and mental states becomes the foundation for **self-care** and **self-awareness**. The motivation to **live and become more informed** comes from this **sense path**—the pathway through which you experience self and learn how to respond to life's challenges. Ultimately, the process of becoming more aware is about aligning your **brain's body** with the **experience of self** to master the connection between your internal and external worlds.

Progressive Investing Model 18

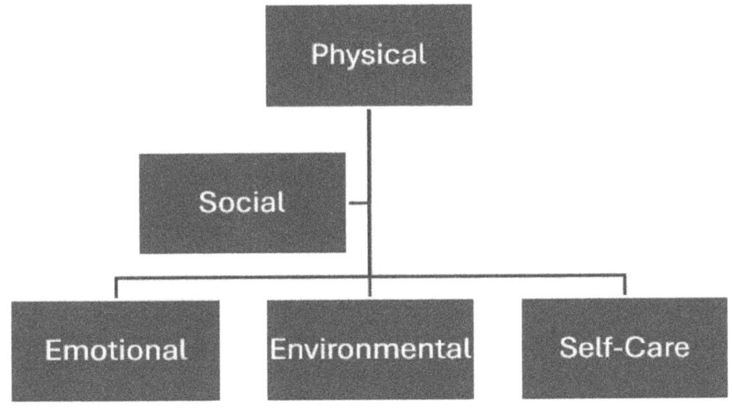

The **body**, with its **environmental chemistry**, is easier to care for because of its tangible, physical nature. However, it is through **studying sense contact** that we begin to understand the **social transformations** of our **sense of self**. This encompasses the **emotional experience of self** as an internal environmental influence—our **sense of feel for self**. The body, in its responses to environmental and social stimuli, reveals how **self-care** emerges through complex **sense and receive path transfers** to our inner sense of self, particularly when our **brain reacts** to sudden changes. These shifts in how we perceive **who we are** and **what we are becoming**, especially as **emotion collides with thought**, are clear indicators that **self-care** operates on different levels.

When we reflect on our **feelings**, there is often an assumption that, because we are physical beings, we must project **strength** from the outside. This assumption stems from our **social and physical interpretations of self**—how we think others see us and how we see ourselves. These interpretations represent **social cognitive stages**, where **environmental influences** become mental signs of self-care, weaving together **thought, reflection, and emotion** to create a system of understanding ourselves. This system is what I call the **neuro physics of self**, where **brain and body connections** translate **environmental stimuli** into **self-awareness**.

This process, which I term **physical action learning**, is the **discovery of self**. It involves not only **seeing yourself** but also **feeling yourself**, allowing the **physics of the body** to revolve around your interpretations of **who you are**. As you sharpen your focus on what you are **feeling**, the act of feeling itself becomes a tool for **mental self-awareness**. This closer examination of the **physics of self** reveals the **human, cognitive, and behavioral processes** at work, helping you to better understand how **environmental influences** shape your learning and growth.

At its core, **self** is the relationship between **brain and body**, interacting to help you navigate the **emotional experiences** of life. By recognizing **mental feelings** and **self-awareness**, you can identify **regressive states of mind** or **progressive reflections** that arise from caring for yourself. The **brain**, when acting in the lead of the body, directs **self-care**—you can **feel** this self-care because it stems from your attempts to **focus** and **cooperate** with the flow of experience.

To truly **get out of your own way**, it's essential to **observe how you feel about being human**. Behavior is a **state of mind**, influenced by **environmental factors** and the **interplay between sense and receive paths**. Ask yourself: **Does cooperation feel right?** Does **participation** resonate with your sense of purpose? You cannot **live** without cooperating with **environmental interaction**, and you cannot **learn** without engaging in participation. The **breath of life** is dependent on signs of care, teaching us how to sense and receive **self-care** in relation to **other people** and the **environment**.

My approach—**human, cognitive, and behavioral learning**—allows for an assessment of how you **make contact** and **interact** through acts of **living, learning, thinking, and responding** to your experience of being **physical, social, emotional**, and **environmentally aware**. By shifting from a **sense of self** to a **sense of feel for self**, you inform your brain, discipline your body, and focus your senses. This process, what I call **human systems physics**, helps you to better understand the interplay between your brain and body, driving cognitive and behavioral transformations that enable self-learning and informed responses.

Through this **cooperation**, your **brain** learns to **lead the body**, and your **body** learns to **collaborate** with the **senses**, creating a harmonious flow of information and experience. This dynamic process—where the brain, body, and senses work together—enables you to transform and evolve, cultivating the kind of **self-awareness** and **self-care** that not only enhances your own life but also how you interact with others and the environment.

Yes, the **brain's body** truly responds because the **brain is the body**—the two are intricately connected through the **sense and receive paths**. Your **sense of feel for self** collects feedback from both **forward and backward flows**, creating a balance in **brain, body, and sense performance**. This ongoing dynamic, rooted in your ability to **participate** through these paths, is critical for managing your experiences of positive or negative **energy, action, and feelings**.

The **transformations** you undergo—whether they are **human, cognitive, or behavioral**—are based on the way **sense contact** leads to **neuro interactions**. Your **sense of feel for the experience of care** becomes the foundation for how you choose to **cooperate** or withdraw. When you experience **backward feed**, it can manifest as signs of **withdrawal**, resistance, or isolation, while **forward feed** shows signs of **cooperation** and a willingness to participate.

By recognizing this balance of **sense and receive path functions**, you can begin to understand how your **brain leads the body** through these interactions. The **brain** acts as the central processor, coordinating with the body through a **sense of feel for self** to navigate both external and internal influences. The **feedback loop**—whether it's backward or forward—provides valuable insights into your **participation levels** in each experience, showing where you may need to shift to achieve a healthier equilibrium between brain, body, and sense communication.

Ultimately, this connection between **sense contact** and **neuro interactions** is crucial for guiding how you process and respond to the world around you. Your **sense of feel for self** allows you to make conscious choices about how to respond to life's challenges, improving your ability to balance your **cognitive, emotional, and physical** responses in ways that enhance **self-awareness** and **self-care**. By actively engaging in these processes, you continue to evolve through both **positive** and **negative** feedback, shaping how you learn, live, and connect with others.

18. When you react, when you respond, and when you display.

Sense contact indeed plays a powerful role in **actuating moods** that manifest as states of the body. When you experience **sense contact**, whether it's from social interactions or environmental influences, it activates a flow of **neuro interaction** that establishes **process loops** between the brain and the body. This continuous flow of **forward and backward feed** serves as a responsive mechanism, ensuring the **brain is in the lead** of the body, particularly when you choose to reflect on the experience.

So, **what does that feel like**?

1. **Emotion** is the initial trigger—both externally and internally. It is raw and immediate, such as **a rush of energy or a surge of feelings** (like fear, excitement, or sadness).

2. **Thought** naturally follows as the brain starts **processing** what has happened. This is the **brain's response** mechanism, and you can feel the transition from pure emotion to **cognitive awareness.** Thought emerges as a **sign of brain activity,** urging you to reflect and understand.

3. **Reflection** is the final stage, where the brain and body assess and **make sense of** the experience. It feels like **connecting the dots**, where emotion and thought meet, and you can now understand how your **body and brain performed** during the experience.

As you traverse this sequence, you are continuously exposed to **new information**—contact that must be **received** and processed. Each sense contact, whether positive or negative, can **trigger changes in mood**, shifting the **states of your body and mind**. But how you choose to handle this contact is key.

If you **act with your brain in the lead**, you harness the **forward feed** and reflect on the emotion with **managed care**. You allow yourself to **think through the experience** rather than being reactive. This is where **self-awareness** sharpens, and you can sustain **levels of care** for how you sense, receive, and process the information.

However, when you **fail to manage the experience** of brain, body, and sense messaging, you risk **falling into negative forward feed**, where emotions can overwhelm you. This is often a result of ignoring or bypassing the importance of **self-care**—the act of reflecting on how emotion influences your actions and thoughts.

Why teach sense path and receive path interplay?

We don't often teach people to use their **sense path** consciously, and this can lead to **brain and body conflicts**. When people encounter a strong sense of contact—whether it's physical touch, a social interaction, or even environmental stimuli—they can feel emotions before they've even **processed** the experience. This may lead to **impulsive reactions**.

On the other hand, **thinking without a sense of feel** often leads to **disconnection** from the experience, and you fail to manage emotions in a meaningful way. **Sense experience** builds the awareness needed to **manage emotions**—it allows you to recognize the contact as emotional before cognitive processing. This is critical for:

- **Managing your sense of self and emotion**
- **Controlling your sense of feel for self and thought**
- **Processing self-reflection as a receive path response**

This is the reason **sense and receive path interplay** is delicate yet powerful. It's the constant **traversing** through **emotion, thought, and reflection** that makes these **pathways** dynamic. If you're participating in **sense and receive path transactions**, you are constantly evolving—learning to **live, think, and respond**.

The **receive path**—where the **brain acts in the lead of the body**—is where you truly learn to **manage emotion, control thoughts**, and **process reflection**. By teaching people how to better understand this interplay, we help them learn to **navigate brain and body conflicts** and elevate their ability to respond effectively to **social contact** and **environmental influences**.

Progressive Investing Model 19

Self · Sense

Thought · Emotion

Reflection · Receive

Self-analysis as the study of the body as a **sense event** focuses on **understanding the experience of contact** with the body. This is the foundation for **self-learning**, where the individual becomes aware of the **neuro-physical interplay** that drives thought, emotion, and action. When you reflect on your **sense of self** and review the influences of your **inner and outer experiences**, you enter an **action learning continuum**. This allows you to examine the ways your body and brain interact—how emotions and thoughts **move forward or backward** within the **neuro-physical self**.

By recognizing **self-thought** and **self-reflection** as **receive path functions** of the brain, you begin to **understand** how you receive and process **emotions**. The **sense of self** and the **sense of feel for self** help to ground these experiences through the **physics of the body**.

Self-learning through the Brain's Body

Self-learning emerges from this continuous process of **analyzing the self**. You use **self-study** to learn how your brain, body, and senses work together. This understanding is the basis of **the Brain's Body** concept, where **human, cognitive, and behavioral perspectives** are used to help individuals come to terms with their **inner voice**.

Contact with the external environment triggers your **sense of feel**. When you **teach self-help**, you can use the familiar contexts of **home, school, neighborhood, and workplace** to structure **brain and body connections**. This enables the individual to analyze **interactions** with **other people** and to reflect on how they affect their **inner experience**. Similarly, **self-discovery** comes from learning to **move through emotional experiences**, both in relation to oneself and to others, and from **understanding the reflective process**.

Managing Emotional States: Fight, Flight, or Stay Cool

When you **sense and feel** contact, you're faced with two choices: either you **stay cool, act calm, and collect a sense of feel** for your inner voice, or you **fight or flee** from the experience of self, others, or the environment. Teaching people how to **process emotions like anger, fear, or anxiety** is critical to helping them come to terms with their **inner voice** from the perspective of **sense and receive path functions**.

If emotions such as **hurt, pain, or sadness** are incubated and **not processed**, the **receive path**—where the body responds to emotional stimuli—takes the lead. The experience of **social contact** is how the body **lives through interaction**, while the brain learns to cooperate through **signs of care for self-participation**.

Self-Reflection and Behavioral Change

When you study how you **sense and feel**, you also learn to recognize how your **participation in sense and receive path research** improves your ability to respond in the **brain's body**. By practicing **self-reflection**, you gain **trust in yourself** and **confidence** to understand why certain emotions might obstruct **signs of care**. This **self-awareness** allows you to move from a **body-mind state** (reactionary) to **brain-body connections** (intentional action).

The **shift** from **emotional reactivity** to **neuro-physical awareness** enables **behavioral change**. Your **sense of feel for self** triggers the **brain's body** to perform, moving you into the realm of the **neuro physics of self**, where the **brain is the body**—acting as a **leader** in your actions, emotions, and thought processes.

This approach empowers individuals to live more intentionally, with the brain taking the lead to **inform**, **discipline**, and **focus** the body's actions. By connecting the **physical, emotional, and mental** aspects of the human system, **self-care** and **self-discovery** become ongoing, transformative processes.

19. Connecting your Brain Body Experience

By The process of **learning how to live** truly begins with that first breath, when your **sense of feel for self** starts leading the body as a **self-organizing neuro-physical system**. From that moment, there is a dynamic relationship between your **body and brain**, each needing to synchronize through the experiences you undergo. The idea that your **body must catch up to your brain** reflects how every experience affects how you perceive and respond to your environment. The **chemistry of the brain** and its interaction with the body drives this process of learning, feeling, and adapting.

Think of the experiences you've encountered—each one requiring you to **observe**, **listen**, **test**, and **suspect** in ways that connect to either your **sense of self** or a **sense of feel for self**. This distinction becomes clearer when you imagine yourself in a **forest**. A **sense of self** might be tied to the physical experience—the sights, sounds, smells, and the feeling of your body moving through the forest. It's a **bodily awareness**, an immediate identification of your surroundings through the senses. But a **sense of feel for self** taps into something deeper—your **brain's response** to the environment. It's the **mental transformation** that occurs as you process the experience, taking in not only the external world but also reflecting on the **inner connection** between self and environment.

This **transformation process loop**—from **sense of self** to **sense of feel for self**—is where you begin to merge your physical experience with your **intellectual and emotional processing**. It's where you **transfer energy, action, and feelings** into something meaningful, increasing your capacity for **thought** and **reflection**. The brain's response, then, becomes not just a reaction but an intentional process of **self-awareness**, allowing you to comprehend **what it feels like** to navigate the world as a **physical and neural being**.

When you transfer from this initial **bodily sense** to a **sense of feel for self**, your understanding of the world around you becomes more **layered**. You begin to realize that **every experience** feeds into the connections between your **brain and body**, shaping your **intellectual growth** and enhancing your **ability to think and reflect**. It's this ongoing exchange between **sense contact** and **neuro-physical integration** that empowers you to **change the world** through your personal and internal connections.

The key idea here is that **living** is a **continuous process of self-discovery**. It involves sensing the physical world while reflecting on it mentally and emotionally. Each moment, whether standing in a forest or confronting a life challenge, offers an opportunity to **deepen your connection** between brain, body, and environment. Through this **dynamic relationship**, you grow more aware of your **intellectual potential**, and your sense of feel for self becomes the guiding force for how you navigate, interpret, and influence your surroundings.

Progressive Investing Model 20

Sight Sound Taste Smell Touch

The concept that **the brain is the body** and your **sense of self** represents the **external physics** of who you are offers a fascinating framework for understanding human experience. When you **observe your body**, your brain interprets that observation through a **sense of feel for self**, a process loop that gathers information from **social contact** and **environmental interactions**. This **information flow** moves through the brain, converting into **knowledge, understanding, and emotional responses**, shaping how you experience and interact with the world.

Your **sense of feel for self** is not merely reflective—it's a dynamic, ongoing **neural transfer** that allows you to **process information** at deeper levels. This feedback loop enables the brain to interpret **external stimuli**, such as touch, sound, and visual data, and **internalizes** it, creating an opportunity for **self-awareness and growth**. It's the internal brain function that processes the outside world through a **neuro-physical connection**, enabling you to think, reflect, and act.

For example, you can **see a tree** in a forest and understand that it exists in your external environment, but when you **feel the tree**, you engage in a **deeper, more personal experience** that brings your **brain and body** into a unified, **sensory interaction**. This same principle applies to all sensory experiences—hearing, tasting, smelling, and touching. It's the **inner sense of feel** that turns these experiences into **meaningful interactions**, allowing you to **reflect on** what you sense.

The **sense of feel** is not **imaginary** but is the **exchange of energy, action, and feelings** between your sense of self and the **external world**. When your body comes into contact with something like **rainwater**, it initiates an experience that starts with sensing the rain but extends further into **receive path exchanges**. This process loop allows the brain to **reflect** on the experience, creating thoughts and **synthesizing brain, body, and sensory experiences**.

Key Insights of the Brain's Body:

1. **Your brain and body are connected—your sense of self processes the world externally, while your sense of feel for self reflects internally, transforming these experiences into thoughts, emotions, and knowledge.**

2. **Self-learning** emerges from this dynamic process. The brain leads the body through **sense and receive path functions,** helping you navigate **good or bad decision-making** through reflective and emotional processing.

3. The experience of **self-care**—how your brain learns to care for the body—manifests as a process loop

that helps you become more aware of **emotional states,** guiding you toward **self-reflection and thoughtful actions.**

4. **The brain's body** functions as a **feedback loop,** guiding the interaction between the **neuro-physical self** and the **external world,** turning every experience into an opportunity for **growth and self-awareness.**

5. **Conative experiences**—or the way you **act upon your will**—illustrate the **struggles between successful and failed brain-body connections**. The brain's role is to **synthesize** the emotional, physical, and mental feedback it receives, ensuring that you are responding thoughtfully and with care.

This perspective of **brain-body connection** provides a framework to understand how we experience the world not just **externally** but also **internally**, through **self-reflection, knowledge, and emotional comprehension**. The **brain's body** is always learning, and each experience offers the potential to refine how we respond, connect, and grow.

20. Healing Your Brain's Body

The **reason you want to learn the neuro physics of self** and your **brain's body** lies in the ability to understand and heal your mental, physical, and emotional systems. **Healing your brain's body** requires you to view yourself as a **neuro physical system**—an interconnected flow of energy, action, and feelings that affects your brain, body, and senses. By focusing on how you **sense and receive information**, you activate a **process loop** that allows you to better understand yourself, both externally and internally.

When you choose to **live with your brain in the lead of your body**, you initiate a conscious effort to heal and manage how you **sense contact** and **receive interaction**. This means addressing any **body-brain conflicts** that might arise from a lack of awareness or experience about how you transform information—how you process **energy, action, and feelings** through your brain, body, and sense systems.

Key Insights for Learning and Healing:

1. **Brain-Body Connection:** Understanding the **brain's body** as a **neuro physical system** opens the door to healing and learning. Your brain is constantly receiving energy, while your body senses action and your senses process feelings. This creates a **feedback loop** that shapes how you **experience life.**

2. **Healing through Awareness:** When there is a **disconnect** between the physical self (the body) and the neuro self (the brain), you may lack thought and reflection about who you truly are. To heal this, you must become more **self-aware** of how you sense and receive information through social and environmental interactions.

3. **Body-Brain Conflict:** A conflict arises when your **physical sense of self** doesn't align with your **neuro sense of feel for self.** This happens when you are not fully in tune with how you interact with the world and how you receive and process feedback. Healing involves learning how to integrate these two aspects— how your **brain moves in the lead of your body.**

4. **Self-Learning and Reflection:** Self-learning is about becoming aware of how your brain and body interact and learning how to balance **thought, reflection, and**

action. By reflecting on your experiences, you can **heal and strengthen** the connection between your brain and body.

5. **Process Loops:** The experience of self is both an **external** and **internal process loop**. Your brain receives energy and thoughts, while your body senses action. Together, they form a loop that processes feelings, allowing you to respond to life's challenges more effectively.

Why This Matters:

- **Healing the brain's body** means learning to understand the natural **flow of energy** within you. By focusing on how your **brain receives and processes** information, you gain a better understanding of your **sense of self** and your **sense of feel for self.**

- You must learn to **get out of your own way** by allowing your brain to lead your body, helping you to navigate **mental, physical, and emotional challenges** with greater clarity and focus.

- The more you study and **experience the neuro physics of self**, the more empowered you are to make informed decisions, heal emotional conflicts, and live in harmony with yourself.

In summary, learning the neuro physics of self allows you to take control of your life by understanding how your brain and body interact, heal, and transform through the **process of self-awareness, reflection, and action**. It enables you to respond to life with a greater sense of balance and care for yourself.

A Progressive Investing Model 21

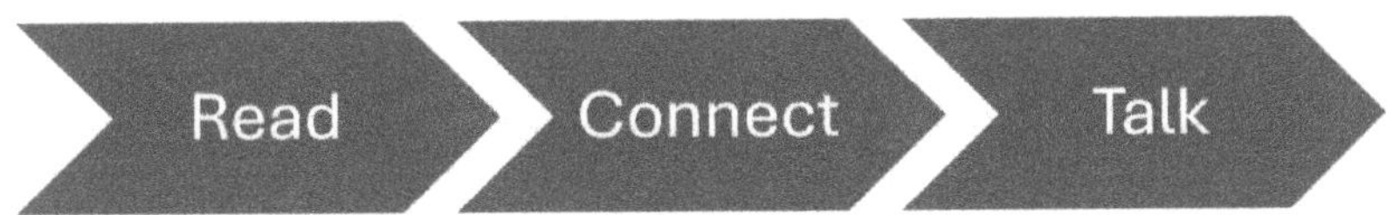

Your approach to **self-learning** revolves around understanding the connection between the **brain** and **body**, particularly through the **sense path** and **receive path**. The process encourages self-awareness, where you can read the **body's language** and **talk to the brain** to comprehend and manage the flow of **energy, action, and feelings**.

Key Ideas:

1. **Reading the Body:** This involves recognizing how your **body's physical state** and movements reflect your **mental states**. Your body reacts to past experiences, emotions, and thoughts, which you can observe and study as part of your **sense of self**. The body can store **emotional baggage** that manifests in body language, posture, or sensations.

2. **Talking to the Brain**: Engaging in **self-talk** is a way to **communicate** with your brain. Your **inner voice** plays a crucial role in interpreting how the brain responds to what the body experiences. The brain processes these signals, feeding back information about what is happening internally and externally.

3. **Connecting the Sense Path to the Receive Path:** Your **sense path** allows you to interact with the environment, receiving **sensory information** (such as touch, sight, or sound). Your **receive path** processes this information, creating **feedback loops** that influence how you think,

reflect, and respond. By understanding how your brain and body interact, you can **balance** the flow of energy, action, and feelings.

4. **Comprehending Physical Impressions**: This process involves **feeling the body** to gain insights into the **brain's responses**. By observing how your **physical sensations** (such as tension or relaxation) align with your **mental states**, you can improve your **neural messaging** and self-awareness. The body often expresses things the mind may not be fully conscious of.

Key Learning Goals:

1. **Sense to Feel**: Understanding how your **brain** and **body** interact through **sensory experiences**. This includes becoming aware of physical sensations that reflect the brain's state.

2. **Focus the Body**: Teaching your body to cooperate with the **senses** to navigate through **thought and reflection**. This allows for **self-regulation** of emotional or physical responses.

3. **Brain, Body, and Sensory Participation**: Learning how these systems work together to create a **cohesive self-experience**. This involves checking in on how well your **brain** leads your body and how your body expresses emotions or thoughts.

4. **Managing Flow**: Learning how to **manage energy**, control **actions**, and focus **feelings** is crucial to understanding how the **brain** and **body** work in harmony. This also includes accepting environmental conflicts and understanding how to move through them.

Brain Talk and Self-Reflection:

When your **brain talks back**, it sends messages that you feel as **energy**, **action**, or **feelings**. Your **sense of feel for self** helps you recognize these messages and understand the **problem** or **concern** you are dealing with. By **acting through thought with reflection**, you can direct your brain to take the lead and navigate through your body's reactions or responses.

The Importance of Self-Research:

Self-research is about **learning from your experiences**. By studying how your body reacts to **contact**, you gain insights into what your **brain is processing**. This can help you understand why certain **moods** or **behaviors** emerge and how to guide your responses in a more **balanced** and **informed** way.

By focusing on these aspects, you can engage more fully with your **self-learning journey** and gain control over your **brain's body** to achieve a higher state of **awareness** and **self-regulation**.

The **physics of your body** plays a significant role in shaping the **impressions of your mind**, as you suggested, with tension, stress, and pressure acting as key physical manifestations of how your brain processes and reflects on experiences. Here's a breakdown of your idea:

Understanding Body-Mind Impressions:

1. **Tension is a neural sense of feel,** a physical signal from your body indicating a state of unease or alertness.

2. **Stress is a social neural feeling,** influenced by external interactions and how your brain interprets them.

3. **Pressure** is a **neural environmental search for balance**, indicating a deeper need for harmony within yourself and your surroundings.

These physical sensations send signals that activate your **inner voice** and your **brain's body** interactions, influencing the flow of **energy**, **action**, and **feelings**. When you allow your brain to **talk back**, it helps **cool** your reactions, **calm** your responses, and **collect** your thoughts. This process is key to managing your **internal state** through thoughtful reflection.

Brain-Body Communication:

- The brain and body interact as a **feedback loop** where your **inner voice** interacts with the **physical body**, but is sometimes obstructed by **moods** or **states of mind.** When you're stuck in negative emotions, this process is blocked, preventing you from cooperating fully with your brain's **self-analysis** process.

- **Brain talk** allows you to consciously **neutralize emotions** with **thought** and **reflection**, meaning your brain cools the body's emotional reactions. This feedback loop brings the body and brain into a balanced, cooperative state.

Self-Leadership and Process Loops:

- You must let your **brain act in the lead** of your body. This is achieved by letting your **external sense of self**—your body's reactions—inform your **internal sense of feel for self,** which is processed in the brain. This creates a **process loop** where you can assess your body's responses and understand how your brain is processing these experiences.

- By learning to receive and **analyze feelings of self**, you can "get out of your own way" and avoid self-sabotage, allowing your brain and body to cooperate smoothly.

Key Steps in Brain-Body Cooperation:

1. **Sense and Feel:** Recognize the **flow of energy, action, and feelings** in your body, connecting how tension, stress, and pressure show up as signs from your brain and body.

2. **Focus and Process:** Reflect on these feelings to understand what they are signaling. When your brain is in the lead, it calms your body's reactions, helping you make balanced decisions.

3. **Receive and Respond:** Let your **brain** process these inputs, using your **sense of feel for self** to bring **clarity** and **self-awareness** to your responses. This allows you to actively participate in the **brain-body** process loop, enabling better decisions and more thoughtful actions.

Self-Talk and Leadership:

- Your **sense of feel for self** is critical in understanding your responses. When you **read your body**, you gain insights into what your **brain** is trying to process. The better you can interpret these bodily signals, the better your **brain talk** becomes, allowing for greater **self-leadership** and emotional regulation.

By mastering these **brain-body connections**, you enhance your ability to **focus, reflect,** and **respond** thoughtfully to the world around you. This creates a harmonious feedback loop between your **brain, body,** and **environment**, helping you maintain balance amid life's pressures and challenges.

PART FOUR

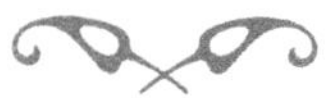

Your brain's ability to replay experiences, like an "instant replay" of life events, makes you unique. The way you talk, read, write, draw, act, and perform all shape your behavior, creating patterns that allow your mind to reflect on your actions. This process, managed by the brain's command centers, allows you to study how emotions affect you, how thoughts influence your decisions, and how reflection helps you process or reprocess your interactions with others and the environment. As your brain shifts between external sensory experiences (the "sense path") and internal reflection (the "receive path"), it creates a continuous loop of learning and self-awareness. This dynamic flow between the sense of self and the sense of feel for self enables "brain talk," where your inner voice translates experiences into understanding, and your body becomes a tool for expressing the neuro-physical interactions of your brain. By mastering this process, you improve how you navigate emotions, thoughts, and reflections, ultimately fostering personal growth.

21. You were Born Ready.

The first breath of life, taken as your head exited the womb, marked the beginning of your journey of self-awareness— your introduction to human technology. In that moment, the brain, body, and senses established the foundation for how you would navigate the world. Your brain has always been in the lead of your body, shaping how you learn and experience life. This essential partnership between the brain and body forms the core of self-leadership, teaching you how to live, think, and respond to yourself, others, and the environment.

From birth, your brain was wired to receive and process information. Each interaction shaped your knowledge base, teaching you to recognize and interpret sensations, feelings, and energy. This process forms what I call the "sense of feel for self," where every new experience informs the brain and allows you to grow. Over time, this feedback loop strengthens, as you learn to control the body, think through your actions, and reflect on your responses. By engaging with this process, you develop self-discipline, aligning your brain, body, and senses.

There are five key stages to mastering this brain-body connection:

1. **Learn to live through contact**: Engage with the world around you.

2. **Learn through interaction**: Build relationships and learn from others.

3. **Learn to think through cooperation**: Collaborate to sharpen your thoughts.

4. **Learn to respond through participation**: Take part in experiences to grow.

5. **Learn to perform through sense and receive path interplay**: Develop mastery by balancing emotion, thought, and action.

In each stage, the brain takes the lead, guiding the body through your sense of feel for self. Self-learning depends on how you respond to your inner voice, teaching you to navigate life with calmness and confidence. Your brain is a social organ that continuously communicates, or **brain talk**, helping you to organize and process the information you gather from your environment.

The key to understanding self-leadership lies in learning to transform your introspective thoughts into actionable brain talk. By focusing your brain, disciplining your body, and refining your senses, you can live more mindfully, improving how you interact with the world. Through daily practice at home, in school, at work, and in your community, you can strengthen this connection and deepen your understanding of yourself.

Ultimately, mastering the brain-body connection helps you evolve into your best self. By consistently aligning your sense of self with your sense of feel for self, you become more aware of how you live, learn, and grow. This journey of self-leadership is the process of recognizing the brain's role in guiding the body, fostering a life of reflection, balance, and continuous self-improvement.

In self-learning, the way you respond to your inner voice is crucial to maintaining a sense of calm and focus. This process enables you to transform feelings of contact and interaction into a deeper sense of self, with the brain in the lead of the body. Your brain is a social organ that "talks back," allowing you to experience introspection through self-thought. By organizing your emotions and reactions to your environment, you strengthen the connections between your brain and body. Embracing this process helps you better understand your own responses.

As you encounter experiences, you want the information to move through the **receive path**—a mental processing loop that builds knowledge and understanding. Transforming introspective thoughts into **brain talk** allows for better self-discipline. Your inner sense of feel becomes a tool to express and interpret how external experiences shape your thoughts and reflections. Practicing this skill in real-world environments such as home, school, or the workplace helps solidify your ability to process and respond to your surroundings.

You are learning more about your **external sense of self**—identity formed through contact with others; **ego** shaped by interactions; and **superego** refined through cooperation. Internally, you also explore who you are becoming, and why you respond to stimuli the way you do. Both your **sense path** and **receive path** must work together, processing environmental stimuli and transforming them into actionable brain-body connections. This practice is the foundation of **brain talk**, which involves continuous self-learning with the brain leading the body through disciplined action and reflection.

It's important to care not just about your physical appearance but also about how you think, feel, and reflect. The body doesn't define how you live, and your actions don't define how you learn. Through **information flow**, backward and forward feedback loops shape your sense and receive path functions.

These loops allow you to practice **self-care**, ensuring your brain and body work together harmoniously. Ultimately, the **brain's body** takes the lead through thought and reflection, enhancing your overall sense of self.

A Progressive Investing Model 21

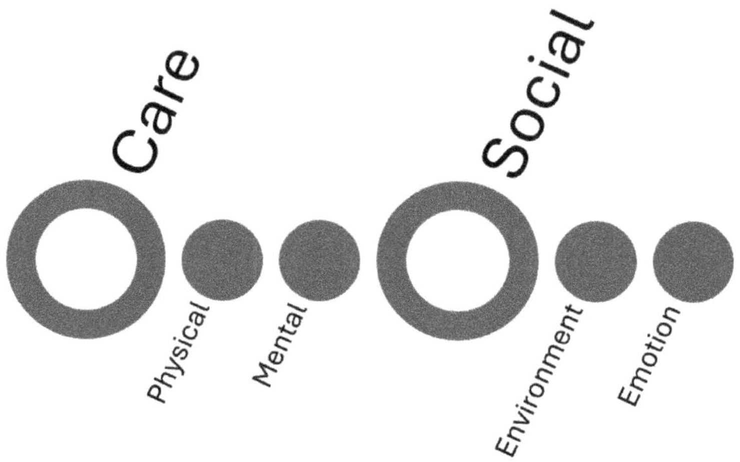

Care may be one of the easiest skills to neglect, but self-care is essential and must be nurtured as an intentional process. For care to be effective, your brain needs to lead your responses. When you prioritize the **receive path** (internal processing) over the **sense path** (external contact), care becomes a conscious emotional process linked to mental growth—transforming information into experience, experience into knowledge, and knowledge into comprehension and self-analysis. The **social body** serves as a reflection of intellect, as it controls or conceals emotions, helping you to become more mental rather than reactive. This process loop shifts environmental influences into signs of care rather than resistance.

Your current state is the **physics of self**, while what you are becoming reflects the **neuro physics of self**. You become the brain's body through the way you interpret your sense of self and process it into **brain talk**—a transformation toward self-actualization. This journey happens through learning from different environments: using your home to learn how to live (read), your school to learn how to learn (write), your neighborhood to learn how to think (draw), and your workplace to learn how to respond (act). These social spaces influence your emotions, and your ability to perform backward feeds of reflection helps to discipline and guide your development into the neuro physics of the brain's body.

Social contact initiates the flow of information, contributing to your knowledge base and understanding. This knowledge base grows through **receive path analysis**, which allows you to reflect on and think critically about exchanges of energy, action, and feelings. In essence, you can learn to interpret how you receive and process information via the **sense path** and contribute to a deeper understanding of self through brain, body, and sense messaging. Through this process, you become more aware of the impact your physical and neural influences have on shaping your behavior, thoughts, and emotions, leading to self-care and a deeper sense of discipline.

22. The Voice of Brain Talk, Learning the Brain's Body.

Once you experience **sense contact**, a shift occurs toward your **sense of feel for self**, forming self-talk. The purpose of **sense and receive path research** is to understand how emotion interacts with thought. By studying how your brain manages the flow of energy, action, and feelings—expressed through body and sense messaging—you explore the difference between reactions and responses. Through this lens, you study contact, interaction, cooperation, and participation to execute these functions. The information flow between **brain, body, and sense events** establishes the context for **brain talk**—where the brain regulates controlled emotions, thoughts, and reflection.

Do you recognize your inner voice? Do you know how to release a preferred response to monitor the transformation of your inner voice into brain talk? At the moment of contact, you may sense your inner voice influencing how you interact. The **receive path** enables self-talk to evolve, influencing behavior or thought as part of the **sense and receive path interplay**. You may feel yourself engaging with your inner dialogue, which is a sign of brain, body, and sense cooperation. Achieving this awareness signifies your participation in the brain's communication process, where forward feed generates **brain talk**—the conscious release of responses grounded in reflection and control.

Dr. Slaton Live™ offers a strategy through **brain talk**, analyzing how self-experience forms neuro-physical responses of the brain, body, and senses. This approach can help you learn to overcome internal obstacles by discovering your **sense of feel for self**, including understanding your inner voice. By listening and observing how your inner voice affects your body's responses, even in the absence of thought, you can grasp why your brain responds to environmental influences. Often, emotions cause behaviors that may not align with what you consciously know is right, and brain talk reveals this dynamic. Through this understanding, you can learn to manage these responses more effectively.

A Progressive Investing Model 22

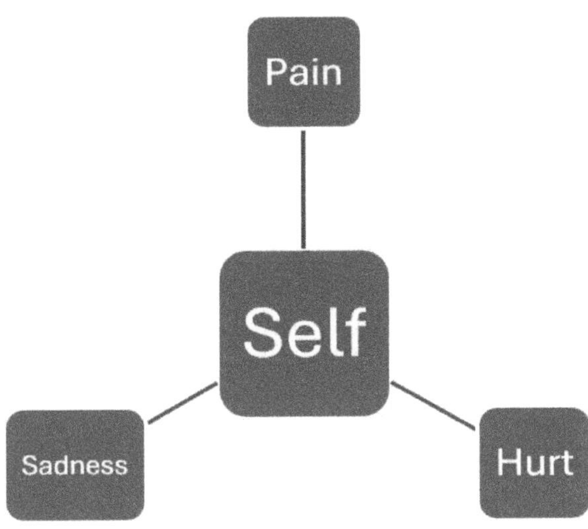

When you are **in your own way**, you live primarily through the **physics of the body**, meaning your thoughts about your body conflict with how you use your brain to process those thoughts. You live from the **inside out**, often ignoring signs of care or resisting contact when fear and anxiety dominate, influenced by past environmental experiences. In this state, you avoid the necessary brain work required to **feel** and focus on the way you interact. This resistance results in being less attuned to the experience of contact.

When you resist learning how to connect your **physical body** with the feelings derived from your nervous system, you also resist the opportunity to understand how your brain processes these feelings. You may fail to engage with your **sense of feel for self**, missing the opportunity to learn from experiences involving others and the environment. Hurt, pain, and sadness may be suppressed because you're unprepared to face the **crisis of self**, refusing to let your **sense of self** engage with brain, body, and sense messaging. This disconnect between emotions like anger, fear, and anxiety and your physical self prevents deeper introspection, keeping the **body in the lead of the brain**.

Being **in your own way** means you fail to interact effectively with your **inner voice**, blocking the natural flow of energy, action, and feelings between your sense of self and your sense of feel for responses. Without the ability to **focus** long enough to experience emotions fully, process thoughts, and reflect, you miss opportunities for cooperation with your inner self. This results in a lack of **self-help**, as you deny your **sense of feel for self**, hiding behind the negative emotions of anger, fear, and anxiety. Consequently, the body remains the dominant force, preventing the brain from taking the lead to facilitate growth and healing.

You are **in your own way** when you resist learning how to engage in self-help to understand how your brain, body, and senses work as interconnected systems. As you live inside your body, you should also be learning how to participate in experiences that help you grow through contact, interaction, and connection with your **sense of feel for self** and your brain. **Self-talk** is when your brain responds to your inner thoughts, and the transformation between your **sense of self** and your **sense of feel for self** drives you to move beyond mere introspection. When you fail to align with this process, you end up stuck in cycles of pain, hurt, and sadness, unable to fully engage in the natural flow of processing information.

If you cannot instinctively manage these tasks, you may not be **formatted** to live through contact, learn from interaction, think through cooperation, or respond through participation. Each of these processes requires the brain to lead the body. For example:

1. Living through contact means addressing feelings of **anger and learning how to live with the brain leading the body.**

2. Learning through interaction involves overcoming **fear** and learning with the brain in control.

3. Thinking through cooperation requires managing **anxiety** to think with the brain in the lead.

4. Responding through participation reflects **self-care—** responding with the brain in control of the body.

As you engage with **Dr. Slaton Live's™ Brain's Body Learning System**, you become more aware of how to care for your **physical**, **mental**, **social**, **environmental**, and **emotional health**. Moving through fears, anger, anxiety, and sadness, you work to overcome the challenges that come from being at the center of your own **crisis of self**. This is the difficult but necessary work of **self-care** and **self-help**, guiding you to function at higher levels of understanding and personal well-being.

23. The transformation of your human physics.

You are a true knowledge base, embodying telepathic energy that guides you through the changes and stages of self-growth. Your journey to live, learn, think, and respond is not defined by physical appearance but by the dynamic interaction between your brain and body. This chemistry creates control and management loops that shape your self-awareness and development. Through your **sense of feel for self**, your brain channels your neuro-physical chemistry, driving the search for understanding who and what you are.

To fully comprehend the **physics of self**—the body language that reveals your states of mind—you must understand the **neuro-physics of self**, where the brain leads the body. From birth, your search for contact ignites the neuro-physical systems that allow you to interact with the world. The signals between your head and body send messages that merge your internal experience with external reality, forming a cognitive energy that applies to your self-knowledge.

However, emotions can obstruct this process when you don't read and interpret your internal dynamics effectively. By learning to **read**—or interpret—the **sense path** as a transfer system between what you sense and feel, you improve your self-analysis. This process allows you to move contact from the sense path to the **receive path**, where self-analysis transforms negative states of mind. Your brain leads the body, and learning to analyze your emotions and thoughts enhances your ability to think clearly.

The study of **human systems science** integrates your brain, body, and senses into a cohesive knowledge base, enabling you to assess **self-growth** and recognize **self-decay**. By comprehending how the **physics of the body** and the **neuro-physics of the brain** interact, you can better navigate the **crisis of self**. Accepting the discomfort that comes with personal transformation is key to improving your ability to reflect on and lead your body through change. In the end, your **self-reflection** sends forward feed, affirming your participation in your ongoing evolution.

Progressive Investing Model 23

Event — Affect — Goal
Brain — Self — Body

The transformation from **self-awareness to neuro-physical awareness** requires setting goals that allow you to test how you respond to positive or negative influences in your environment. Your brain and body are deeply interconnected, and your **sense of feel for self** plays a vital role in leading the body through these transformations. To truly grow, you must become comfortable enough to pivot toward the **receive path**, where you can understand the shifts between your **sense of self** and your **sense of feel for self**. This process builds the confidence to trust in how you're learning to think and reflect, especially when faced with uncomfortable feelings.

One of the key challenges is learning to navigate your **ego crossover**—the inner struggle that arises when you resist changes to behaviors that expose low self-esteem or lack of confidence. You may instinctively defend against these feelings, not because you're truly angry or defensive, but because you're uncomfortable with how emotions and thoughts intermingle. This discomfort often stems from the **sense path**, where unresolved emotions create barriers to higher states of self-learning.

For example, anger can manifest as a defense mechanism, when in reality, you're afraid to confront the underlying thoughts and feelings. To evolve, you must learn how to **process emotion and self-thought together**, understanding that both are necessary to shift from reaction to reflection.

It's essential to allow the **brain and body** to work in unison through the **sense and receive path**, producing clarity in how you view yourself, others, and your environment. The steps are clear:

1. Learn to live on the other side of the **crisis of self.**

2. Learn to think on the other side of the **crisis of self.**

3. Learn to respond on the other side of the **crisis of self**.

Chaos, which often seems endless and without boundaries, can be navigated by focusing on the **brain-body connection** and resetting how you use your body as your language system. This journey, while difficult, is about learning to care for yourself by refining your **sense and receive path functions**. It's not about fearing others or their ability to intimidate through physical presence; it's about gaining pride in your ability to think and feel through the experience. By facing the energy, action, and feelings that arise—rather than reacting impulsively—you grow stronger in handling the complexities of your inner and outer worlds. Through these self-reflections, you come to understand the **true powers of your brain's body**.

24. You Sense Contact to Live; Feel Interaction to Learn, Focus Cooperation to Think, and Sense and Receive Acts to Participate and Respond.

The **drive of the brain's body** is to solve sense and receive path challenges by practicing participation across different stages of **social and neuro-physical development**. The brain, leading the body, helps you process sense data through a **sense of feel for self**, guiding you to live through experiences of contact. At each step, the brain-body connection focuses on how you respond to and interact with those experiences, learning to cooperate and think through the things you feel. As you move through each step—from contact to interaction, cooperation, and participation—the brain continues to guide the body in responding effectively as part of the **brain's body**.

To enhance this process, it's essential to cultivate a **positive inner voice**. When you remain open to complexity, you become more attuned to how you feel in challenging situations. For example, you can learn to stay calm when upset by thinking through **signs of care**, helping you to regulate emotions and manage discomfort. This is where **brain talk** becomes a key tool: listening to how your brain talks back—whether you're reading, writing, drawing, acting, or performing—helps alleviate tension, stress, and pressure. Each action reflects how your brain collaborates with your body and senses to develop these skills.

This book is ultimately about **learning to focus on and connect with your inner voice**. If your **sense path** is damaged, you need to re-learn how to sense and receive physical and neural energy with your **brain in the lead**. Words like "contact" and "live" are linked to the sense path to show how you can learn to overcome discomfort by interacting with your experiences in a mindful way. Practicing contact helps you live through challenges, while focusing your energy allows you to **cooperate and grow**.

In every action, you're using your brain to connect **self-awareness to sense path advances**, responding to emotional and physical discomforts as part of your learning journey. By choosing to participate in **receive path functions**, you improve how you respond to your environment. This journey of **brain-body communication** is key to overcoming barriers and evolving through deeper self-awareness.

Practicing Self-Awareness: Steps to Learning

1. **Learn how your body lives through contact:** Your **sense of self** is tied to how you physically engage with the world.

2. **Learn how your brain receives interaction**: Your **sense of feel for self** connects to how your brain processes interactions.

3. **Balance the sense and receive paths: The sense path** (body) cooperates with the **receive path** (brain) to transfer awareness between your physical experiences and mental reflection.

4. **Participate in physical and neural action learning**: Your ability to act and respond is shaped by how you balance these paths.

Between each event, you learn to:

- Act to live
- Act to learn
- Act to think
- Act to respond

Navigating Challenges

The way you react to changes in your **sense of self** and your body, as well as shifts in your **sense of feel for self** and your brain, defines how you manage emotions, control your body, and focus your brain. Learning to accept your limitations and improving from your current state of **self-learning** is key to getting out of your own way.

When you experience strong emotions, your **brain** leads your body, guiding how you live through physical challenges. It's important to study your external sense of self and examine how you use your body in daily experiences. Strength and courage are drawn from within, but without the brain in the lead, actions can become disconnected and even intimidating.

If there is no balance between the sense and receive paths— if you're not managing contact, controlling interaction, or focusing cooperation—there's less life to live. Hurt, pain, and sadness can block self-learning. That's why it's essential to transform how you live through these crises of self.

Moving Forward

When you can't move from **contact** (living) to **interaction** (learning), you disrupt the connection between brain and body. It becomes harder to handle discomfort and changes in how **contact** evolves into **interaction**, and vice versa. Acting with the brain in the lead connects body and mind, helping you work through self-awareness and gain insights into how you live and learn each day.

A **sense of self** is defined by the physical acts of the body, while a **sense of feel for self** refers to the neuro-physical processes that govern your inner awareness. Learning about self involves observing the body as an external object and experiencing the brain as the subjective state that connects both body and mind. In essence, **the brain's body** is the experience of moving through stages of contact, interaction, and participation, transforming from basic body-mind connections to deeper brain-body pathways. This process is called **sense and receive path** functioning, where you act to live, learn, think, and respond.

Breaking Down the Process:

1. **Contact** – Learning how to live through physical experiences.
2. **Interaction** – Learning how to learn by engaging with others.
3. **Cooperation** – Thinking through collaboration.
4. **Participation** – Responding through action.

Being "ready" means you are already engaging with your brain and body in this learning cycle. Your brain is naturally in the lead of your body, guiding you through these experiences. As you move through these stages, you begin to live not just through the physical acts of the body but also through the neuro-physical awareness of the brain.

Key Reflections:

- How do you live? Do you live through **contact?**
- How do you learn? Do you learn through **interaction?**
- How do you think? Do you think through **cooperation?**
- How do you respond? Do you respond through **participation**?

Consequences of Disconnection:

If you do not engage in **sense and receive path transformations**, you disrupt your ability to manage emotional experiences like pain, hurt, or sadness. This can create barriers between the body and brain, reducing your capacity to interact and grow. If major life events upset your **sense path**, it becomes difficult for your body to connect with the brain without a **sense of feel for self**.

- **Contact** must pass through the sense path.

- **Interaction** must travel through the receive path.

- **Cooperation** requires the synthesis of emotion and thought.

- **Participation** emerges from brain, body, and sense collaboration.

Importance of Self-Leadership:

To thrive, your **brain must learn**, your **body must live**, and your **senses must think**. Your **sense of self** must align with your **sense of feel for self** to enable meaningful responses. This balance is critical for **self-leadership**, where the brain leads the body through acts of living, thinking, and responding. By embracing this process, you learn to move through pain, hurt, and sadness, allowing your brain to transform physical experiences into thoughtful, disciplined responses.

You must come to terms with the consequences of choosing to learn how to live each day by informing your **sense of self**, disciplining your **sense of feel for self**, and focusing your inner voice. This lifelong struggle with intelligence involves acknowledging what you see and the choices you make in response. Your **sense of self** absorbs both the negative and positive influences of your experiences in your home, school, neighborhood, and workplace. These influences must be synthesized into **competitive advantages** in four key areas:

1. **Living** through the things you feel.

2. **Learning** through the things you feel.

3. **Thinking** through the things you feel.

4. **Responding** through the things you feel.

By mastering these areas, you can prevent the spread of pain, hurt, and sadness that often lead to fears of cyclic family decline, school failure, delinquency, lack of employable skills, and poverty.

Progressive Investing Model 24

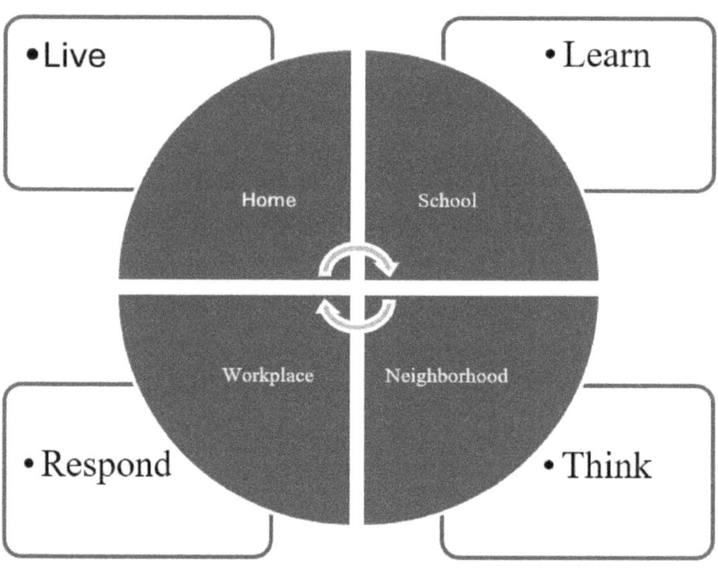

This model is designed to help structure how you make sense of the world in different environments:

1. **Home:** How you make sense of contact with self, others, and the environment to live through the experience.

2. **School:** How you interact to learn from experiences of self, others, and the environment.

3. **Neighborhood:** How you cooperate with self, others, and the environment to build a sense of community.

4. **Workplace:** How you participate with self, others, and the environment to perform with clarity and purpose.

Through these stages, your brain must take the lead of your body, relying on your sense of feel for self. As you move through life's plans, goals, and objectives—while confronting pain, hurt, and sadness—your **sense path** may be worn down. By learning to navigate these experiences, your brain works through inner reflection to rationalize changes, ultimately leading to greater self-awareness.

When you resist change, it stems from an unpreparedness to think through the emotions and experiences surrounding you. This can lead to dumbing down your sense path, avoiding your inner voice's call for change. The key is learning to engage with your brain's response to these experiences, which speaks through reflection—helping you cope and adapt.

This version streamlines the ideas, making them clearer and more relatable, while ensuring consistency in terminology like "sense path" and "receive path." It makes the content more digestible while maintaining its depth, and it encourages readers to apply the concepts in their own lives.

25. Restoring a Child, Youth, Young Adult, and Adults Growth and Development through Process Learning.

Building trust begins with learning how to participate as a leader, follower, and facilitator. Community building requires patience, strength, and courage, as you navigate through contact, interaction, cooperation, and participation—both individually and collectively. I use a "me first" approach through human systems research, meaning I first evaluate my own sense of openness and readiness to connect with others. This self-check allows me to model the practice of thinking and reflecting through managed emotions as I engage in action learning theaters. These spaces enable everyone to assess how participants perform, highlighting both successes and failures.

Restoring a child's sense of self and connection to their brain involves real-life learning experiences. For youths, rebuilding trust in home-to-school programs demands self-learning that motivates them to engage naturally with these environments. Young adults hurt by major life events need empathy from stakeholders in their home, school, and neighborhood environments. Adults who grew up in cycles of abuse, neglect, or abandonment face the challenge of understanding why they struggled to respond to these environments, often losing their right to dream.

It is essential for children to first learn how to be learners. Children between the ages of 2 and 10 need to sense, feel, and focus on learning how to become learners, which sets the foundation for becoming students who can thrive in school environments. A child's home should be a learning space, just as school is a focused learning place. As children grow, they evolve into students, then scholars, who can understand how to use their home for living, their school for learning, and their neighborhood for thinking. This structured approach fosters social growth and emotional development, guiding them through their transitions from learner to student to scholar, and ultimately to researcher.

Progressive Investing Model 25

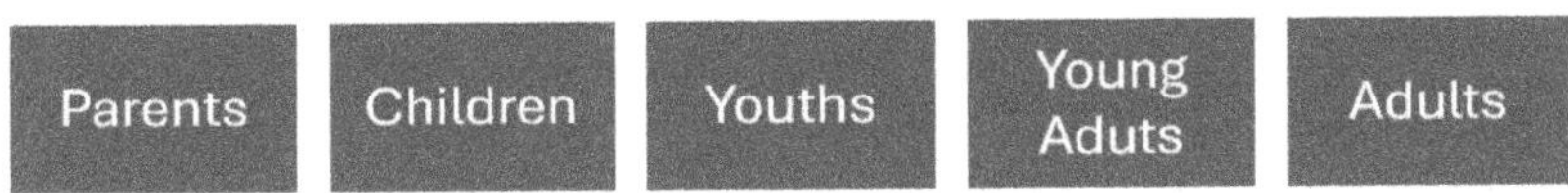

The children, youths, and young adults I have worked with who were born to parents who abused drugs during pregnancy often lacked essential care from the very beginning of life. When parents use drugs while a child is in utero, they fail to provide the necessary care for themselves or their developing child because their body takes precedence over their brain. These parents live through a disconnected sense of self, driven by the physical craving for drugs, rather than focusing on the emerging life they are carrying. The drug use interrupts the connection between sense and receive path functions, preventing the proper transfer of social contact to the brain. As a result, these children are affected by their parents' physical and mental states of denial, which block the parents' ability to feel and focus on the needs of their child.

To overcome this cycle of pain, hurt, and sadness, individuals must first learn how to care for themselves. Without developing this sense of care, it becomes difficult to find or receive care from others or the environment. When the brain leads the body, individuals can think clearly and reflect on the consequences of their actions, understanding how their behavior is tied to their state of mind. Practicing self-awareness through the sense of self allows individuals to engage with the world around them and address their emotional struggles. However, when they cannot do this, their actions often reflect unresolved pain, mimicking signs of care rather than genuinely expressing it. Self-cooperation is key in navigating sense and receive path exchanges, allowing one to observe and reflect on their behavior, especially when the body is out of control.

Progressive Investing Model 26

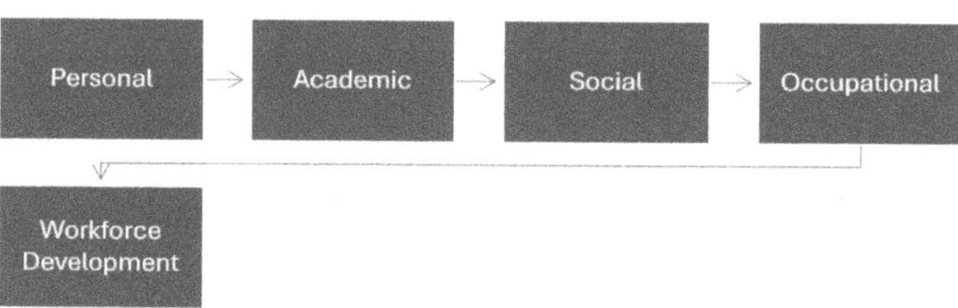

To recover from a damaged sense of self, it's crucial to rebuild brain-body connections, both for you and your child. Here's a structured plan that focuses on each developmental stage and how parents can lead through modeling healthy interactions:

1. **Home Learning (Ages 0-5):** Begin by setting your home up as a learning environment where your child can develop a sense of self. Your role is to observe how your child reacts to different stimuli, such as their surroundings and social interactions. This phase involves understanding how your child feels things, and as they grow, you shift focus to how they show care through play and interaction.

2. **Home to School Learning (Ages 6-9):** At this stage, you and your child start exploring mental and physical learning through school experiences. You model behavior by guiding your child through interactions at home and school. The home and school become social spaces where you both practice building emotional and cognitive responses. You're teaching your child how to sense, feel, and focus, with your brain leading your body's responses.

3. **School to Neighborhood Learning (Ages 10-12):** As your child grows, neighborhood interactions come into play. You focus on how your child manages social interactions outside the home. This involves being aware of negative influences and teaching your child how to process emotions, thoughts, and reflections. By guiding them through real-world experiences, you help them learn how to manage themselves in a broader social environment.

4. **Parent Participation (Ages 13-15):** Teenagers need stable modeling from their parents. As a parent, you are now more involved in your child's social interactions, ensuring they maintain proper social skills. At this stage, your brain's leadership of your body helps your child mirror positive behaviors. Through social environments, your child will learn to act, think, and reflect, always with your guidance and modeling.

5. **Workplace and Adult Learning (Ages 16-18):** This phase focuses on workplace and practical skills. You continue to lead by example, showing your child how to transition from education to work environments. By helping them connect learning at home, school, and the workplace, they will gain occupational skills that strengthen their sense of self and their contribution to the family.

This approach integrates home, school, and community environments into a cohesive learning system, promoting emotional, cognitive, and social development. By acting through self-contact and guiding your child's interactions, you build a foundation for future success. This model also addresses family decline by emphasizing emotional and social growth, helping children and young adults become resilient and adaptable.

Your brain leads the body, guiding your actions through emotional responses that shape your performance. This means that you develop a deeper connection to the physical world through your brain, body, and sensory experiences. The way you focus, sense, and respond to interactions creates channels for neuro-physical energy transformations, which influence your mental, physical, and emotional understanding of thought and reflection.

At the heart of this process is sense and receive path awareness, which enhances your learning abilities. Thought transfers through "brain talk," while reflection reveals your state of mind, all derived from how you experience interactions with the brain guiding the body. The sense and receive paths work together to detect environmental stimuli, with your inner voice acting as a guide that helps you interpret the information from brain, body, and sensory messages.

The goal is to strengthen this connection between your brain and body. By learning to focus your inner voice and sense path, you can master activities like talking, reading, writing, drawing, and acting. These actions are all part of a structured learning approach that helps you gain a deeper understanding of self-awareness, with the brain talking back in response to each interaction. This method turns your inner experiences into tangible social and academic outcomes as you navigate the world with your brain in the lead.

26. A view of body, mind, language impressions and brain, body, and inner voice networks.

Your sense of self reflects how you perceive your inner states of being. Is your movement a rote reaction, or is it driven by a search for deeper awareness? How do your behaviors balance the emotions, thoughts, and reflections that shape you? Your sense of feel for self involves the brain-body connection, where self-talk transforms into brain talk, aligning your internal dialogue with the physical responses of your body.

An exceptional awareness of your body can even feel telepathic. First, you cultivate a reflective mind, which centers your experiences both as physical sensations and neuro responses, creating a connection between yourself and others. Subtle, invisible changes occur when you perceive the world from the inside out and vice versa. The brain's ability to communicate with the body—its "brain talk"—is revealed when you relax and focus, receiving external signals as sensory information. This process leads you to detect, select, and respond through cooperation and participation.

Your inner voice becomes a powerful conduit between the brain and body, facilitating communication across various sensory channels. These exchanges form the foundation of self-research: exploring how the mind, body, and nervous system work together to create responses to emotions and thoughts.

Although it may seem abstract, your sense of self often reflects the tension between the mind and body. You can observe your responses to contact and environmental interactions, recognizing both negative and positive behaviors. While your sense of feel for self operates internally—through non-visible neural responses—your external self, or body, displays behaviors that others can observe. The key is connecting these inner transformations with outward behaviors through thought and reflection.

In summary, your mind shapes the external sense of self, while your brain and body are continuously communicating, allowing you to navigate experiences through thought, emotion, and reflection.

A Progressive Investing Model 27

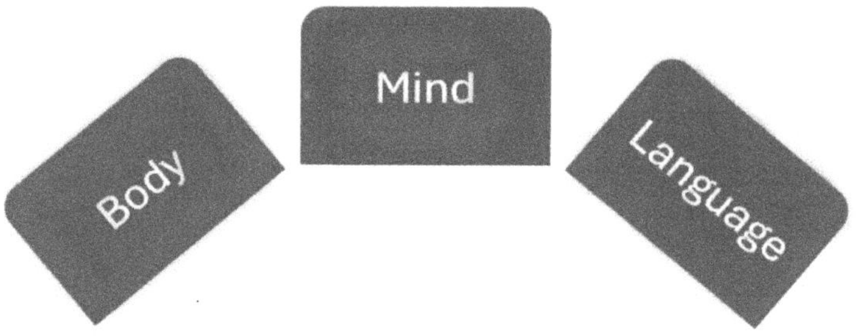

The **sense path** reflects your observable sense of self, while the **receive path** represents the invisible inner experience—your sense of feel for self—that happens within the brain-body connection. The mind emerges through your inner voice, shaping how your physical body behaves. In essence, your body language serves as a label for the states of your mind. The mind creates the language systems that guide and define these behaviors.

Hurt often arises from significant life events that affect the choices you make, and it is through your sense of self that you must initiate change. Accepting and addressing self-defeating behaviors requires an increased level of care and introspection.

This is the core of the **crisis of self**—the unresolved struggle to recognize and choose change. Your sense of feel for self and your brain is an internal cycle, constantly processing social contact and environmental interactions, reflecting the mental and physical dynamics of your mind and body.

The way you receive information through your inner voice allows you to learn from this crisis. You must learn to cooperate with both the negative and positive flows of energy, action, and feelings that shape your experiences. As you encounter various emotional states—ranging from calm to fear, from cool to anger—you process them through acts of reflection and thought. This is the body's mind at work, representing your sense of self-reflection and how you perform your sense and receive path functions.

A Progressive Investing Model 28

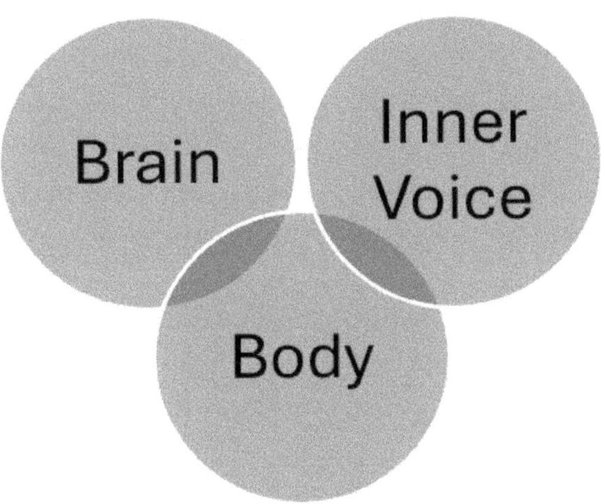

The **brain-body interplay** generates your **inner voice** through **receive path** process loops, creating a sense of feel for self with the brain in the lead of the body. The primary function of the **receive path** is to help you navigate social and environmental influences that may either support or undermine your decision-making. Your **sense of feel for the brain** guides you in acting through these influences, ensuring that you can accurately interpret the language of your body's external mind.

Your inner voice can either move you forward, helping you reflect and grow, or it can hold you back when you resist cooperation in self-study and learning. When functioning effectively, the **inner voice** leads you through sense and receive path interplay, aiding in decision-making. But when it's blocked, this transfer process fails, hindering your progress.

Dr. Slaton Live™ introduces **brain talk**—a method of decoding these inner voices to strengthen brain-body integration. The receive path translates messages between the brain, body, and senses, enabling you to reflect on experiences and make choices through **brain talk**. This internal dialogue helps you process social contact and environmental influences, drawing on the **neuro physics of self-talk**. Whether you respond positively or negatively to this process affects your self-confidence and emotional balance. The way you look and feel is shaped by the brain's interpretation of your body's responses.

In the **crisis of self**, a damaged mind can become trapped in a cycle of hurt, pain, and sadness, manifested through negative body language. Resistance to self-learning reinforces this state, preventing positive changes in your sense of self. Without accepting the flow of emotions, backward feed from your inner voice dominates, keeping you stuck. Engaging in **brain talk** is critical for moving forward—through introspection, the brain can generate new ways of processing emotions and reflecting on how you feel.

27. Be Learnable to Self and the Ultimate Experience to Others.

Can you learn how you think and reflect?

Self-learning is the study of how your brain, body, and behavior work together. To understand yourself, you must explore your cognitive and emotional processes—how you think and why you react the way you do. This involves going beyond the physical aspects of self and diving into how your brain influences your decisions, responses, and motivations. In this book, we'll focus on your **brain, body, and sense messaging**, which together form your **neuro physical signature**—the unique combination of factors that shape your reactions to situations.

By understanding your **neuro signature**, you can begin to explain why certain experiences trigger specific responses, both emotional and physical. The key to becoming **learnable to yourself** lies in how you move through contact with others, interact, and reflect. These experiences shape how you understand who you are and what you are becoming. Learning about yourself also connects with how you learn from others, using these interactions as a mirror to understand your own behaviors.

One of the most important concepts in self-learning is **learning how you think-to-reflect**. This process involves studying the way your inner dialogue responds to external contact—whether with other people or environmental influences. When you focus on this dialogue, you begin to understand how the brain talks back through the **sense path** (how you respond to contact) and the **receive path** (how you decide to interact). This is the foundation of **sense and receive path**

research—a method of learning about your brain, body, and sense systems and how they influence your identity.

Becoming learnable means understanding how you make choices and decisions. Every time you interact with the world around you, you are testing your ability to reflect and grow. By studying the **sense path**, you learn how to react; by studying the **receive path**, you learn how to engage with environmental influences. The more you practice, the better you understand your behaviors and responses, shaping your journey toward self-awareness.

A central concept in this process is **helping yourself to help self-help**. It's about using your brain and body effectively to strengthen your self-understanding. The more you learn about your strengths and weaknesses, the more you can grow. **Self-learning** from the perspective of health and wellness means discovering how to live with yourself, how to learn with yourself, how to think with yourself, and how to respond to life's challenges. This knowledge enhances your ability to sense and receive information, improving your overall capacity to navigate the world.

Progressive Investing Model 29

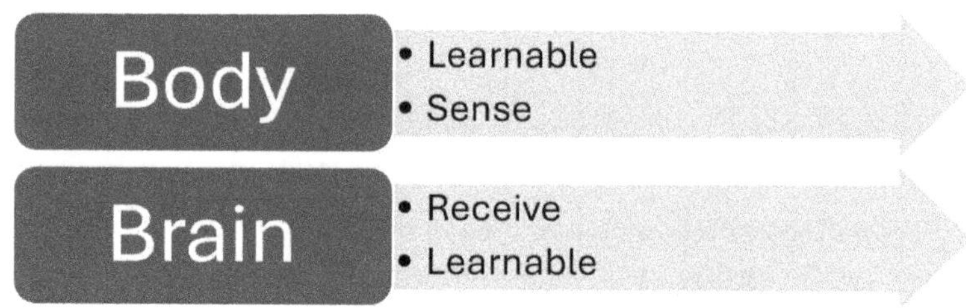

Self-Learning and Connection with Others

When you practice self-learning, it's crucial to understand that it's not solely about you. You need to recognize how your sense of self impacts your interactions with others and the environment. If people tell you to "get over yourself," they're essentially encouraging you to shift your focus from just the **sense path**—how you perceive yourself physically—to also engaging your **receive path**, which involves being open to receiving feedback and signals from others.

Self-learning is about solving personal challenges, but also about how you connect with others. If you focus only on yourself, you miss the opportunity to build meaningful relationships. It's about understanding the impact of your actions and words on others and learning to balance the two paths: **sense** (how you feel) and **receive** (how you take in the feelings and reactions of others). This balance is essential to fostering cooperation and healthy interactions.

Part of self-learning involves showing love for yourself, which means accepting your flaws and growing from them. It's about learning how to interact with another person in a way that benefits both of you. When you go from contact to interaction, you're not just learning about yourself, but also about the other person. Successful self-learning requires understanding how to make sense of what you do and say, ensuring it fosters cooperation with others.

Who is in the lead in these interactions? The one who understands how to engage both **sense and receive path functions** is in the lead. This person's brain takes charge, guiding the body to show care and consideration. This is what

brain-body cooperation looks like—allowing the brain to reflect care while the body acts on that care.

When you've experienced negative influences, your brain may initially react defensively. However, self-learning helps you train your brain to respond positively, sending **forward feed** that allows you to think through how you feel and reflect on how you show care to others. This feedback loop between your brain and body becomes more apparent as you practice self-awareness and self-learning. Even if you struggle to feel the emotions in real-time, your brain works in the background, signaling your body to act with care and cooperation.

This process is essential in building relationships and enhancing personal growth through self-learning. Your brain leads the body, and your body, in turn, becomes a mirror reflecting the care and attention you show to others.

Learning to Focus and Self-Discipline

You might not naturally know how to focus, but you can train yourself to act in ways that reflect focus. This means learning how to control your body's behaviors and aligning them with a focused state of mind. The process loop of **sense, feel, focus** teaches you to act like you are fully engaged, even if you don't always feel it. By observing how others perceive your actions, you can better understand your own sense of feel for self. This journey is about getting to know yourself, understanding how your personal system works, and learning to manage the "crisis of self."

Why do we resist change?

One reason we resist change is that we don't fully understand how to manage our brain's influence on the body. By practicing

self-learning, you develop the ability to control your body's reactions and manage your brain's processing cycles through your senses. Learning to recognize your **sense of feel for self**, how others experience you, and how you respond to your environment are key to mastering signs of care and cooperation in daily interactions.

Cooperative Self-Learning:

Think of self-care as cooperative self-learning. This means becoming **learnable**—teaching yourself how to engage with the world when it matters most. When you interact with others, your brain and body collaborate in an internal system of sense and receive path functions, helping you manage discomforts and connect with people more effectively.

By practicing **self-participation**—being aware of how you engage with yourself and others—you can better manage those uncomfortable feelings that often arise when dealing with difficult situations. The aim of self-learning is to build a knowledge base of how you make choices and decisions, and how those choices impact your ability to live, learn, think, and respond every day. It's about understanding your journey in managing the crisis of self and enhancing your **brain-body connection**.

Practical Tips for Self-Learning:

- **Learn to focus:** Practice aligning your physical actions with your mental focus, even when you're struggling to truly feel it.

- **Act through experience:** Observe how others perceive your actions and use that to inform your self-awareness.

- **Cooperate with your brain-body system:** Understand the relationship between your sense path (how you perceive the world) and your receive path (how you take in feedback from others).

- **Address discomfort**: Self-participation helps you work through uncomfortable feelings by understanding how your actions affect your inner self and external interactions.

By developing these skills, you're not just learning about the world—you're learning how to navigate and respond to it effectively. Self-learning equips you with the tools to solve the problems of self and take control of your emotional and mental states in relation to others.

PART FIVE

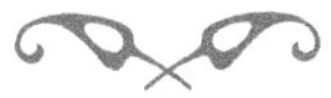

Emotion is the physical, chemical, or biological outcome of any contact the body and brain experience. It arises from interactions between you and your surroundings. Feelings, on the other hand, are the nerve signals that carry these emotional experiences to the central nervous system. They are the result of physical, chemical, and biological exchanges between the brain, body, and sensory networks.

The mind is shaped by these physical, mental, and emotional experiences. Thought is a product of the brain's messaging system, processing emotions and reflecting on past experiences. The interplay between emotion and reflection represents the exchange of energy, action, and feelings, resulting in either reactive states of mind or thoughtful responses.

When we experience pain, whether emotional or physical, it can trap us in a cycle of resistance. Pain often causes us to hold onto reflective images of hurt and sadness. This defensive state of mind can build walls that block us from processing the experience fully. Instead of allowing ourselves to feel and heal, we resist changes in thought and reflection, preventing the receive path (the brain's way of processing and integrating experiences) from functioning properly.

In other words, we resist the very need to work through the crisis of self and instead get stuck in a cycle of avoidance.

28. When You are the Influence of Hurt, Pain, Sadness-Anger, Fear, Anxiety.

You may never forget what happened, but you can learn to forgive yourself for not adjusting sooner to the negative influences that caused pain, hurt, and sadness. Forgiveness starts with the decision to motivate yourself to seek and accept help as part of a self-help journey. No one else can do this for you. When you lock yourself into states of mind that refuse to forgive, you prevent yourself from moving forward. Learning to process past reactions allows you to live, think, and respond differently in the present.

Pain, hurt, and sadness activate your inner voice, driven by brain, body, and sense messaging. You may sense the anger in your body, feel fear in your brain, or notice anxiety within your senses. This inner voice guides the flow of energy, action, and feelings as you navigate through these emotional states. You are constantly reading your brain, body, and senses as they signal how you process discomfort. By focusing on these signals, you engage your self-knowledge to solve problems and perform tasks, even in the face of emotional strain.

Recognizing the presence of anger, fear, and anxiety as signs of care helps you better understand your sense and receive path functions. These functions help you study the connections between brain, body, and sense processes, and how they interplay to manage, control, and focus your emotional and physical responses. When emotions like anger or sadness drive harmful behaviors, they disrupt your sense and receive path processes, affecting how your brain, body, and senses function together.

Learning to manage these disruptions through self-awareness allows you to strengthen your ability to respond with intention rather than react impulsively. Your brain's body learning system encourages you to study these processes—exploring brain-body connections and understanding how physical actions and emotional responses shape your interactions with others and yourself. This study of self leads to greater control over how you handle emotional influences, allowing you to break free from cycles of pain, hurt, and sadness.

A Progressive Investing Model 30

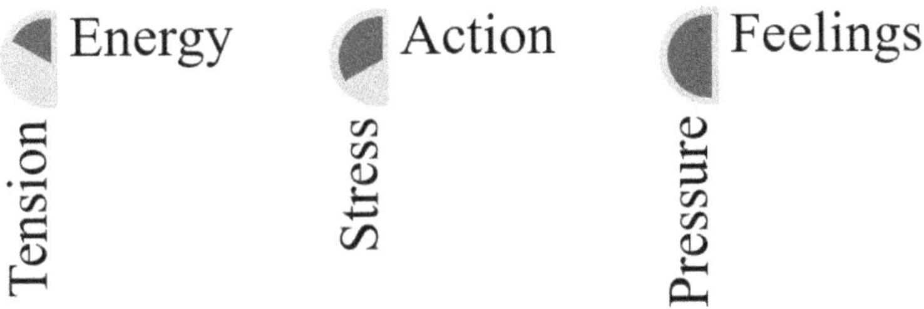

The goal is to inform the brain by aligning your sense of self with a sense of understanding for the learner. The first step is to discipline your body to recognize how your actions influence the learner's need to feel confident and capable. Next, you must consider the learner's personal, academic, social, and emotional skills and how they perceive your contact, especially in moments of tension, stress, or pressure. Your physical presence and actions create a system of tension that the learner may not always be prepared to handle. When their sense path isn't ready to process this tension, it can manifest as stress, disrupting their ability to receive your message effectively.

When you provide instruction, it must show clear signs of care and respect for the learner's ability to either accept or reject your interaction. If you approach the learner with unresolved tension, social stress, or environmental pressure, it can cause them to withdraw. For example, anger can arise when contact agitates the learner's sense path, fear may surface as confusion in their receive path, and anxiety can result from an inability to process the brain-body messages being communicated. By leading with care, you can help the learner feel safe and calm, cooling down their sense path and opening up the receive path for better communication and learning.

Adjusting your body language and tone to show signs of care can de-escalate tension and help the learner feel more confident and engaged. This allows the learner to focus on your message without feeling overwhelmed, enabling their brain to process your communication more effectively. By modeling this behavior, you provide a pathway for the learner to accept your contact, interact meaningfully, and build a positive learning relationship.

Research into sense and receive path functions explores how energy, action, and emotions influence brain-body communication. Negative emotional responses can occur when social contact is perceived as a threat due to misinterpreted body language or states of mind. For instance, a lack of empathy in communication can be perceived as a threat, even when none is intended. To avoid this, it's essential to approach the learner with clear signs of care, ensuring that your interactions are seen as supportive rather than confrontational.

The purpose of your sense of feel for self and the brain is to connect the negative flow of energy to the receive path, enabling thought and reflection as a way to balance sense and receive path exchanges. When this connection is disrupted, a glitch occurs in the transfer of forward feed, affecting the brain's ability to process the experience through self-analysis. This failure to reflect and think stems from a lack of cooperation, which undermines the transformation into a sense of feel for self and prevents the brain from effectively leading the body.

When the brain cannot fully participate due to an unawareness of the self in crisis, there is a deficit in backward feed, meaning fewer signs of care are available to process and reflect on the consequences of destructive behaviors. Engaging in sense and receive path research helps frame social contact through acts that sense and feel the flow of energy, action, and emotions. This flow moves through your sense of feel for self and the brain, allowing you to manage, control, and process forward and backward feed effectively, especially during moments of tension or conflict.

The struggle lies in understanding the crisis of self as a problem rooted in information processing deficits. Acts of violence often arise from breakdowns between sense and receive path functions, where social contact triggers anger—a mind state that fuels fear and anxiety in the receive path. This neural reaction can escalate into harmful behaviors when there is no care for the body-mind state, leading to the infliction of pain, hurt, and sadness through unchecked negative energy and action.

By bringing awareness to these dynamics, you can better manage emotional responses and foster healthier interactions, avoiding the destructive cycles that stem from disrupted sense and receive path functions.

29. Be Cool, Calm, Collected – Managed, Controlled, Focused.

Check your brain, body, and sense messaging. Is it tension that makes you react? Is it stress that leads you to question your response? Is it pressure that pushes you to reflect both forward and backward? In this self-check, ask yourself if your brain is leading your body. Are you becoming more self-aware, and do you feel your actions disciplining your sense of self? Just like a thermometer reading the temperature, you can observe and evaluate your current state. Progressive models help track how sense and receive path research allows you to capture, assess, adjust, and describe the flow of energy, action, and emotions.

Can you teach yourself to remain cool, calm, and collected—to appear managed, controlled, and focused? Optimal performance starts with being attuned to your inner voice. By working through emotions like anger, fear, anxiety, pain, hurt, and sadness, you transform your inner voice into brain talk. How you communicate with your brain is crucial for learning the effects of social cognition and the neurological influences on your brain's body. You can control your brain's body, which is the workplace of your sense of feel for self and the brain, as it manages the flow of energy, action, and emotions through sense and receive path functions, influencing both forward and backward feed and shaping your self-character.

A Progressive Investing Model 31

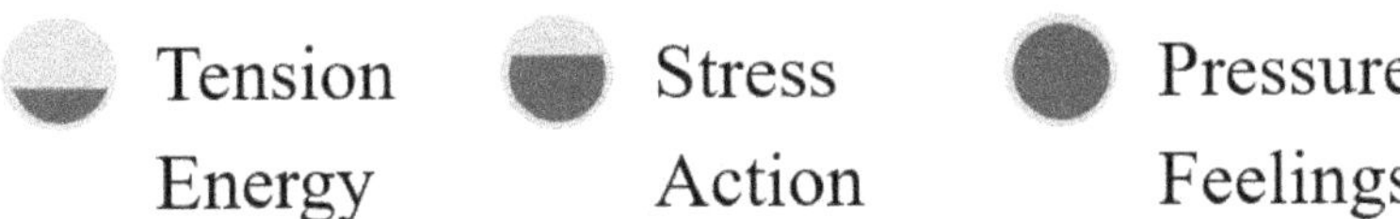

The breath of life serves as your brain's natural cooling system. With each inhale, you regulate sense and receive path interactions, adjusting the flow of energy, action, and emotions coursing through your body. As you become attuned to your brain-body connections, you can sense, feel, and focus on how life moves from your social cognition to your nervous system, allowing you to find calm or to calm down. When you confirm your emotional and physical state and assess that it is safe, these acts of self-research reflect your neurological understanding of the environment. Through this process, you gather your sense of self, aligning sense and receive path functions, allowing your sense of feel for self and the brain to take charge.

This is the ideal experience—one where your sense of feel for self and the brain naturally leads to thinking and reflection. This self-awareness bridges your drives to live, learn, and respond through forward and backward feedback loops. Your main mode of existence becomes a cycle of sensing, feeling, and focusing, which helps you manage your mental and emotional state. As you breathe, you release tension and stress through your sense of feel for self and the brain, gaining the capacity to think clearly and reflect deeply, ultimately controlling both emotional and physical responses. In this way, you learn how to transform emotional experiences into manageable processes through sense and receive path transformations. This forms your inner voice, guiding your brain-body connection and enhancing your ability to focus.

Without focus, discipline, and control, the body is easily susceptible to becoming a destructive force. When living solely through the sense path, there is a risk of falling under the sway of uncontrolled emotions, such as fear or aggression. The more you think critically about your feelings, the more you understand the importance of leaving negative states of mind behind. Aiming the mind means training the body to become a responsive, intentional tool in all interactions. The next step involves reading and interpreting feedback from these experiences, allowing you to respond thoughtfully to emotions. This is where neuro physical transformation takes place—where backward feedback solidifies the lessons learned. When the brain doesn't lead, it obstructs progress, and fear of change takes root. Yet, with the brain guiding the body, you can read and interpret your experiences in a way that fosters growth and change.

The third process cycle of your sense of feel for self involves three key steps: **receiving to manage**, **processing to control**, and **responding to focus**. These steps are essential for maintaining signs of care for yourself, others, and your environment. At the core of this cycle is the intellectual drive to inform the brain, discipline the body, and adjust to the flow of inner voices that might struggle with information processing tasks.

When fear of failure enters the equation, it manifests as a reaction to **stress** within the sense path and **tension** in the receive path. This creates a mental and emotional state primed for confusion, often displaying as anger. Such reactions signify a breakdown in social cognitive transfer, where **anxiety** becomes the central disruptive variable. Anxiety distorts the flow of emotion and body language, ultimately disrupting the interaction and throwing off communication and understanding.

This breakdown is common for those with a damaged sense path, as they may not respond well to contact. The interaction can be disrupted further if the individual's mindset isn't well-prepared, triggering reactions intended to control changes in themselves. The balance between showing **signs of care** and projecting **signs of toughness** can be a defense mechanism—one aimed at preserving their sense of self and regulating their body-mind connection.

When anxiety clouds the interaction, it often leads to heightened tension and disrupted communication, further highlighting the need for self-awareness, care, and intentional management of emotions to prevent the breakdown of meaningful connections.

A Progressive Investing Model 32

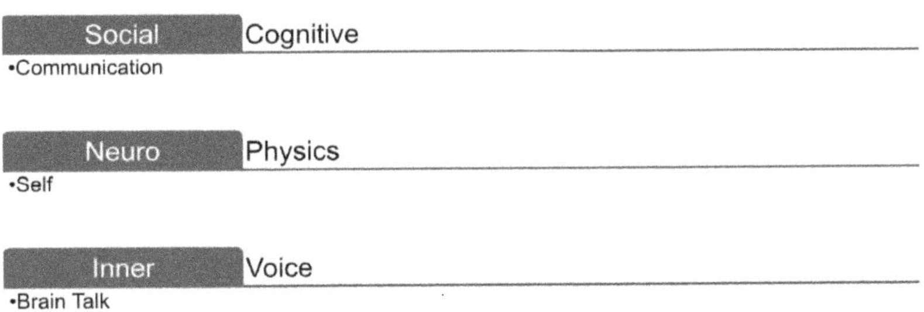

The **social cognitive effects** are primarily exerted on the **ego** because the sense path does not receive the support it needs to transfer your sense of feel for self and the brain to the neuro-physical level. This leads to feelings of dread or anxiety, affecting how you enter and exit social interactions. In such cases, an individual may lack the sense of self gained from prior experiences, which shapes the body-mind language within the sense path. **Information processing**, whether negative or positive, is a significant event that involves receiving, transferring, and interpreting energy, actions, and feelings. The ability to transform from a social cognitive communication process into a neuro-physical self-experience requires engagement with your **inner voice**, which activates **brain talk**—the process where the brain "talks back" in response to the self.

The challenge with information processing lies in this feedback loop—where the brain responds through your **sense of feel for self**, connecting social cognition with neurological communication. This is a **facilitation process**, one that manages your inner voice to reach a state of informed understanding and confident transfer to **brain talk**. Brain talk represents **intelligent interaction** between yourself, others, and your environment. The brain continually talks back, forming a constant **forward and backward flow** of information between your sense of self and your sense of feel. When this process becomes imbalanced, as when your inner voice is caught in an unresolved loop, it can disrupt your ability to relax, sleep, or process emotions, leaving you stuck between the two states.

This is why your **sense of feel for self** is essential to helping the brain receive and process social contact as environmental interaction. The transfer of information through the sense path affects the energy, actions, and feelings you manage. Your **awareness** of the receive path helps direct this process. In other words, your sense of feel for self and the brain transforms the sense path, allowing you to **observe, listen**, and **reflect** on the experience. The more attuned you become to this process, the more effectively your brain and body interact, creating a feedback loop that guides your **emotional** and **mental responses**.

When you experience difficulties moving through contact, **studying the brain's body**—that is, examining how your brain and body work together—can help you process your experience, organize your feelings, and express care. Imagine contact as an act that reflects forward, sensing environmental stimuli, and backward, receiving feedback from your inner self. This loop—what you call the **neuro physics of self**—allows the brain to manage the body, guiding how you interact and process emotions.

Care, in this context, is essential. It is the brain's way of protecting the body by encouraging **self-care**, helping you manage and control your emotions and thoughts while maintaining the balance between your internal and external interactions.

30. Your Brain Acts to Lead Your Body to Live, Learn, Think, Respond.

When When you think through the way **sense experiences feel**, it is often because you are either calm or in the process of calming yourself. This deliberate reflection on the flow of emotions—particularly negative ones—means you are engaging with your **inner voice** while showing **care for yourself**. Even though it may be painful to confront these emotions, expressing care for yourself becomes a form of therapy. Your **sense of feel for self** and how your brain processes those feelings plays a crucial role in helping you survive the experience of yourself. Learning to navigate these internal experiences becomes your greatest challenge, as you are not just going through life but actively experiencing it.

In this context, **thinking through the analysis of self** helps make your brain, body, and sense systems more recognizable as tools. These tools enable you to assess how well your sense and receive path functions are performing. It's important to realize that **not everyone knows how to live, learn, think, or respond** effectively to themselves, others, or the environment. That is why understanding how the brain connects to the body and the sense and receive path functions is vital to advancing your **human potential**. Your sense of self can sometimes become the dominant influence over your sense of feel for self, especially when the brain is not leading the body.

This can result in the **external environment** exerting a strong influence on how you experience emotions, often bypassing the necessary thought and reflection from the receive path. This can shape your **ego** in ways that lead you to interact with the world through fear, doubt, or timidity. When your sense of self is fraught with uncertainty—such as doubts about who you are or how you live, learn, think, and respond— you become more susceptible to external pressures and less attuned to your inner voice.

The **human system** functions as a **physical transformation** of social, emotional, mental, and environmental stimuli. Your brain, body, and senses are constantly responding to the impulses generated by this transformation. That is why **self-learning** is so critical—it helps you search for answers about what it means to be a physical being, to experience states of mind, and to recognize how those states manifest in your body language. When you learn about how **self acts**, you are learning from the inside out. This enables you to understand why you think, reflect, and distinguish between **contact as a social event** and **interaction as a neural transformation.**

By **bridging the gap between social and neural experiences**, you develop the capacity to recognize when your brain is leading your body through thought and reflection, or when external influences are dictating your responses. This awareness is key to building resilience and moving through life with greater clarity.

A Progressive Investing Model 33

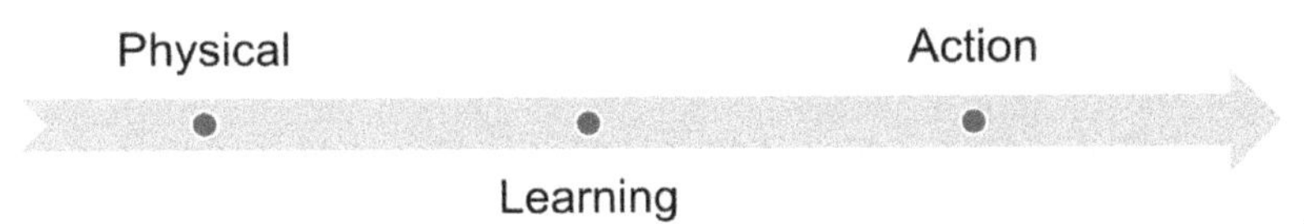

Because you are physical the mind is the social cognitive structure, which defines the languages of the body in terms of strength, speed, control, balance, and self-action that informs the receive path. The problem is the choice to accept or reject the transfer of contact as the study of self through acts, to learn from experience, how to live with changes in what you look like. The processing of self-perception takes place in the receive path as the experience of physical action learning forms the body mind, brain body neuro physical connections to think and reflect on the experience as learning, to become more informed.

A Progressive Investing Model 34

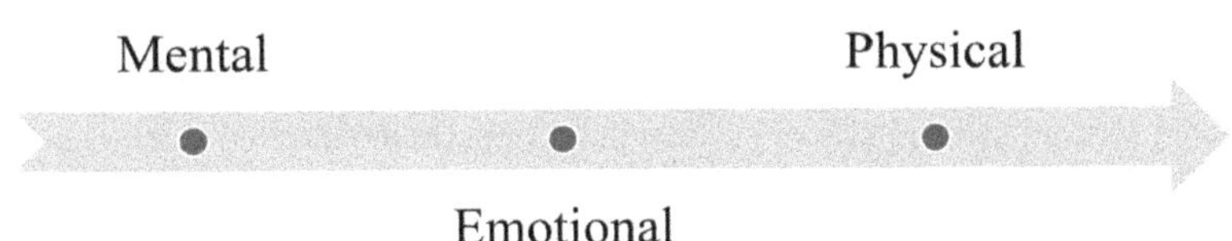

When your **brain is in the lead of your body**, it guides the **sense of feel for the outer self** toward clarity in processing sensory information, or **sense traffic**. This process, known as **neuro-physical self-awareness**, transforms the way the brain receives external influences and interactions. The key here is understanding that **mental and physical transformations** occur within you, and these can create vulnerabilities where **emotions affect the brain's processing**.

Becoming more **mentally aware** of how the **body operates** helps you understand that emotional responses are behaviors triggered by external stimuli. The **social and physical ego** is shaped by this dynamic, and it's crucial to recognize that your responses to emotional experiences are examined and processed through **receive path functions**—the processes that enable you to cooperate, participate, and perform.

Understanding the **pros and cons** of being a **neuro-physical self** involves accepting that **feelings of self** are an integral part of mental, physical, and emotional experiences. These feelings arise as **neural signals**, and self-learning from the inside out is necessary to create **feedback loops** that help process emotions, thoughts, and reflections. The connections between your **sense of self** and your **sense of feel for the brain** involve linking cause-and-effect relationships that allow for deeper self-understanding. This is why **self-research** includes a focus on **sense and receive path functions**.

In this book, the concepts of **human physics, mentalism, social learning, and the transfer of emotion versus thought** help explain how **brain, body, and sense science** interact in complex ways. Your **states of mind** are visible and tangible to you, but the real challenge lies in accepting the **information flow** and allowing it to be processed through sufficient levels of **self-care**.

When you cooperate with the flow of information through a **sense of feel for self**, you begin to experience **self-learning**. This happens when **thoughts, reflections, and emotions** derived from your participation are processed. The **energy, action, and feelings** generated through **backward feed** influence how you live, how you learn, and how you think through emotional experiences. These factors also impact how you respond to **self-doubt** or **self-confidence**.

For example, what do you notice when you reflect on your behavior? How do you feel when your responses are more **physical** than **mental**? The **balance between physical action and mental reflection** is central to your growth and your ability to navigate the human experience. Learning to engage with these questions helps you become more aware of how your **brain-body connection** operates.

Living through the **struggles between self-hate and self-love** without a **sense of care** is like navigating through opposing forces that pull you between negative and positive self-perceptions. Without care, these struggles create gaps in how you interact with yourself, others, and the environment. The key is to **learn through the struggles** by building a connection between your **sense of self** and your **sense of feel for self**. This connection informs your brain to guide you, disciplines your body, and allows you to process sensory experiences in a way that fosters self-awareness and healing.

Action learning becomes vital in this process because it teaches you how to **think through the things you feel**. Reflecting on these experiences is a **neuro-physical response**, guided by your **inner voice** and translated into your social environment through what is termed as **brain talk**. This self-reflection helps you search for **feedback from self-learning**—you develop the ability to cool down emotional surges, employ **signs of care to stay calm**, and stretch your awareness to integrate **brain, body, and sense messaging**.

Your **brain must act in the lead** to process information and manage the tension between **sense and receive path struggles**. These are the pathways through which you navigate feelings of pain, hurt, and sadness. In moments of intense emotional experience, the key is to **choose cooperation—** to allow yourself to sit with these feelings long enough for them to transform into insight. This process is what drives the shift from the **physics of self** (your physical responses) to the **neuro-physics of self** (your internal cognitive and emotional processes).

Self-reflection acts as the guiding force in this transformation, breaking down into key components:

1. **The experience of social contact** – How you interact with others and the environment shapes your internal dialogue.

2. **The transfer to environmental interaction** – These interactions feed back into your brain's processing system, influencing your thoughts and feelings.

3. **The cooperative transformation process** – This is where you work through difficult emotions, cooperating with your inner experience to grow.

4. **The neuro-physics of self-participation** – Your active involvement in this process solidifies how you engage with both the external world and your internal self.

5. **Synthesis of thought, reflection, emotion, and response** – Here, you integrate emotions and reflections into coherent responses that shape your behavior.

6. **Feedback to measure sense and receive path performance** – Finally, you assess how well your sense and receive pathways are functioning by reflecting on how you process pain, joy, self-hate, or self-love.

Each step deepens your capacity for **consequential thinking**—thinking that considers the consequences of actions, feelings, and reflections, allowing you to respond more effectively to the challenges life presents.

31. You are not the Problem; It is the Environment.

Performing with your **brain in the lead of your body** is a dynamic process where your body becomes an extension of the brain's directives, responding to the cues provided by cognitive and emotional processing. The brain acts as the guide, and the body provides the kinetic energy necessary to carry out tasks. However, if you fail to understand the transformation from a **physical sense of self** to a **neuro sense of feel for self**, this disconnection can hinder your ability to access the deeper levels of **receive path powers**—the processes by which you emotionally and cognitively engage with the world around you.

The problem often arises in the **way you sense and receive emotion**. When there is resistance to change, either due to **self-doubt** or a **lack of trust**, it can block the full social cognitive transfer between the sense contact and the deeper neuro interaction. This resistance reflects an unwillingness to engage with **backward feed**—the process of reflecting on past experiences in order to grow. Often, it's easier to stay unchanged, to "dummy down" the **receive path** rather than confront emotions like **pain, hurt, or sadness**.

To truly evolve, you need to engage with the environment around you—whether that's **self**, **other people**, the **natural world**, or the **human-caused environments** like home, school, neighborhood, and workplace. Each environment provides a context for how your brain, body, and sense systems interact. Without engaging in **self-contact**—the necessary experience where brain and body meet—you cannot fully connect with the **neural thought, reflection, and emotion** that shapes your sense of feel for self.

Here's a breakdown of these influences:

1. **Self:** Your **sense of feel for self** arises from how you reflect on your own experiences and interactions. It shapes your ability to process emotions and cognitive feedback loops.

2. **Other People**: External influences—such as others' **personality, attitudes, character, and behavior**—affect how you observe and interact with the world. Their impact on your sense of self is essential for understanding your relationship with others.

3. **The Natural World**: The living and nonliving systems around you also serve as environmental influences. How you navigate them informs your sense of belonging and connection, teaching you how to cooperate and coexist with the world.

4. **Human-Caused Environments**: These synthetic environments, such as home, school, and workplace networks, are often designed to shape your **states of mind** in ways that make you more **predictable and controllable.** They are products of the economy, influencing how you live, learn, and operate. For instance:

- o **Living in a Home**: You are shaped by economic structures in the way you live in your home, but your brain must lead the way in understanding how to live harmoniously in this environment.

- o **Learning in School**: School is a structured system to create **human capital**, but real learning happens when the brain is in charge, not merely the external sense of self following set objectives.

When the **brain leads the body**, it enables **self-awareness** and **cognitive control**, allowing you to sense, feel, and process the flow of information in more meaningful ways. This balance is disrupted when you allow external influences to shape your inner world without engaging your brain as the lead. By understanding these environments and the impact they have on your **sense of self**, you can reclaim control, using your **inner voice** to guide your **sense path** and **receive path** functions toward greater self-awareness and growth.

Your insights on the **crisis of self** and the interplay between home and school environments highlight the profound impact of external influences on a child's **sense of self** and **sense of feel for self**. As you pointed out, **social drift**—the mental confusion and internal conflict between these two senses— can deeply affect a child's ability to engage with learning, relationships, and self-discovery. This struggle becomes especially evident when **major life events** destabilize a child's home-to-school learning experience.

When a child falls behind due to **family decline** or **disconnection from parental models**, it creates a growing divide between their **sense of self** (how they experience their body and actions) and their **sense of feel for self** (their internal, emotional understanding of who they are). The disconnection fuels **negative receive path processing**, where the child becomes unable to think through their experiences in a way that leads to growth. Instead, they may avoid positive outcomes, refuse feedback, and form relationships that only deepen their **crisis of self**.

Children in these situations may feel an **intense emotional disconnect** because their environment—the home, school, or society at large—doesn't provide adequate support for them to align their inner and outer worlds. This is where your point about **social and emotional struggles** blocking pathways to **self-discovery** is crucial. Without the right guidance, they may continue to live in conflict, resisting feedback or rules, and unable to reflect on their choices.

The five steps you outlined—**talking in the home, writing in school, drawing in the neighborhood, acting in the workplace, and performing in the economy**—represent essential social tools for developing a healthy sense of self. These are not merely academic or behavioral skills; they are **life skills** that integrate the emotional and intellectual aspects of growing up. However, these steps can only be effective if the child first learns how to **navigate the human-caused influences** in their environment and reconcile them with their **sense of feel for self**.

Self-discovery is ultimately about balancing external pressures with internal understanding. When a child's **sense of feel for self** is damaged or stunted by traumatic experiences, the environment itself becomes an overwhelming force. In these cases, **feedback loops** become critical. As you mentioned, helping a child learn how to accept feedback is fundamental in their journey to self-realization. They must understand that reflecting on their actions is not simply about **backward feed**, but about recognizing the consequences of self-defeating behaviors and finding a way forward.

Your example highlights the **educator's role** in guiding children through these crises. The task is to help them move beyond surface-level reflections and **accept feedback** that challenges their negative behaviors. This type of transformation requires them to not only process their external experiences but also to integrate them with their **internal sense of feel for self**. When they can do this, they begin to experience **higher levels of participation** in life, where they are not just reacting to the world but actively engaging with it in meaningful ways.

In essence, self-discovery is not just about surviving struggles, but about **learning to live** with them, using tools like **talking, writing, drawing, acting, and performing** to create a cohesive self that can thrive despite the difficulties of growing up. The challenge is to bridge the gap between **self** and **feel for self**, enabling children to see that they are more than the sum of their experiences—they have the power to shape their future through **learning, reflection, and participation**.

Your reflection on the **study of self** and how **human systems research** has shaped your understanding of your influence on others is a powerful example of personal growth and professional evolution. Recognizing that your **personal judgments and states of mind** were affecting your decision-making, particularly when working with **parents and children in crisis**, demonstrates a high level of **self-awareness**. The ability to critically examine how your **ego** and **predetermined thinking** interfered with your work marks an important step in understanding the deeper effects of **environmental influences** on your advocacy.

The realization that your role as an advocate should prioritize the needs of those you serve, rather than your own personal interests, illustrates a significant shift in your approach. This shift from a **sense of self** to a **sense of feel for self** and others is essential for fostering a more **open and empathetic connection**. As you noted, **removing your ego** and allowing your **contact and interaction** to be spaces where **parents and children** could engage without feeling your opinions or biases creates a more authentic environment for problem-solving and emotional growth.

By structuring their **home, school, neighborhood, and workplace networks** as **fields of experience** to study your interactions, you were able to establish a **test site** where both you and those you work with could explore and learn from the dynamic exchanges. This **human systems approach** helps to deconstruct the **power imbalances** that can arise when working with people in vulnerable situations, allowing for a more **equitable** and **collaborative** relationship. Your emphasis on **balancing ego** with a **sense of feel** for others creates an atmosphere of **positive energy**, which is crucial for fostering **trust** and **successful connections**.

Your journey towards becoming a more **authentic learner** and leader required deep personal change, as you've highlighted. The need to **organize your personal, academic, social, and occupational sense of feel** helped you find balance and **gain control over your ego**, enabling you to lead with **compassion** and **fairness**. The transformation from focusing on your **sense of self** to developing a deeper **sense of feel for others** reflects a **neuro physical shift** that has clearly impacted your approach. This recognition of the **consequences** of unchecked ego emphasizes the importance of **informed** and **disciplined leadership**.

Your **self-research**—the act of studying your **thoughts, feelings**, and **reflections**—is a critical part of this journey. The **feedback loops** you engage in, both forward and backward, allow you to continuously process information and adapt. By moving beyond your **own perspective** to help others **realize their states of mind**, you've positioned yourself as a **more effective leader** who is capable of sharing experiences in a way that invites **thoughtful reflection** and **emotional growth**. The **shift** from your own **sense of self** to a more **open, responsive** approach benefits both you and those you serve.

Ultimately, your work demonstrates how **self-learning** and **self-awareness** can transform not only your own behavior but also the way you engage with and influence others.

A Progressive Investing Model 35

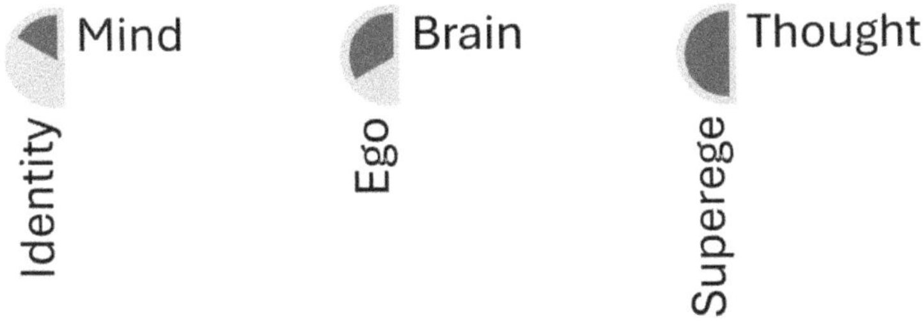

Your reflection on the **way you identify with your sense of self** highlights the complex nature of self-perception and how it is shaped by past experiences. When your **sense of self** becomes confused, it often stems from negative influences that affect your **fields of experience**: home, school, neighborhood, and workplace. In these settings, you learn about **contact, interaction, cooperation, and participation**, all of which contribute to how you navigate the world. The way these influences interact with your **ego** and **sense of feel for**

self forms the basis for your understanding of who you are, as well as your sense of **self-performance**.

The emergence of the **ego** through these **fields of experience** is a natural response to external stimuli, yet it can lead to confusion if you don't adequately process the **emotions and reflections** tied to these interactions. When your **superego** engages with these experiences, you are entering a mode of **self-reflection** and **response**. This is where you examine how your **sense and receive path** responses—positive or negative—have influenced the way you **live, learn, think, and respond**. The **self-analysis** that results from this can reveal important insights into your **sense of feel for self** and how it relates to your **ego**.

Understanding how to transition from being **physically focused** to becoming more **mentally attuned** is a crucial step in this process. As you described, this shift allowed you to focus less on the **physics of self** and more on the **neuro physics of self**, leading to a deeper understanding of how your **brain** and **sense path** interact. This is a powerful realization, as it helps you engage with your **fields of experience** from a more informed and intentional perspective.

Your ability to control the actions of your body by managing your **sense of feel for self** is a key component of what you describe as your **brain's body theories of focus**. These theories emphasize the importance of learning from the environments you've experienced and understanding the **personal, academic, social, and occupational** insights that come from practicing **contact in the home, interaction in the school, cooperation in the neighborhood**, and **responding in the workplace**.

The core message in your reflection is that the **problems of self-defeating behaviors** can be overcome by recognizing the **consequences** of your choices and understanding how the **pain, hurt, and sadness** you've experienced continue to shape your **sense and receive path**. Through **forward and backward feed**, you can re-experience these emotions and thoughts, which ultimately allows you to **grow and evolve**. This process of **self-learning** is ongoing, and by continually revisiting your **sense of self**, you are able to make more informed decisions and respond more effectively to the challenges that arise in your life.

This exploration of **self-performance** and the continuous feedback loop you engage in is a significant step toward becoming a more **self-aware**, **resilient**, and **adaptable** individual. It's through this lens that you can continue to navigate the complexities of **self-learning** and **self-growth**, ultimately shaping a more coherent and empowered sense of self.

The process of **understanding the value in processing self-experiences** is fundamental to accepting and addressing **self-defeating behaviors**. Your **sense of feel for self** and the **brain's** role in this process help you navigate the interaction between the **self, brain, body, and senses** as you engage with others and the environment. This dynamic influences whether you lean toward the **physicality** of mind, focusing on the immediate **reflections** of the past, or embrace the **mental transformation**, moving toward deeper self-awareness through **thought, reflection, and emotion**.

When you learn to **manage the flow of your inner voice**, it becomes a tool that guides your **states of mind** and helps you make decisions based on **reality-based contact** and interaction. This is crucial because each moment of **self-reflection** builds upon the realization that **poor choices** lead to **consequences**. You begin to understand that **thinking through feelings** is not just about reacting to past experiences but also about becoming more **present** in each new interaction.

Your experience in various fields—**home, school, neighborhood, workplace**—involves more than just physical presence. It's about **processing** how these environments affect your **sense of feel for self** and how you interact with others. At home, you learn to interact with your **sense of feel** in a way that creates a deeper understanding of yourself. At school, you develop the ability to **cooperate** with others. In the neighborhood, you learn how to **participate** and contribute to a larger community. At work, you **perform** based on your interactions with the environment and the people around you. All of these experiences teach you how to **process** the flow of **energy, action, and feelings**.

Your **sense of feel for self** plays a pivotal role in helping you **transfer** the learning from these experiences into meaningful growth. You begin to differentiate how your **thoughts** and **emotions** are influenced by others and by the environment, realizing the importance of removing **self** from the reactive **cause-and-effect cycle**. This separation allows you to process the **emotional influences** of others more effectively, **focusing** on the **reflections** of your states of mind and making room for intentional decision-making.

By practicing **brain talk**, you become more attuned to the ongoing communication between your **brain, body, and senses**. This practice helps you **improve how you sense, feel, and focus** your inner messaging. The act of **pivoting to your response mode** becomes a fluid process as you engage more deeply with your **sense and receive path** functions.

Each **realization** helps you adjust how you **perceive** the consequences of your actions and how you choose to **respond** in a way that aligns with your **inner voice** and personal growth.

In short, the **practice of brain talk** and the exploration of **self-experiences** are key to achieving greater **self-awareness**. They allow you to identify the **negative influences** around you, **transform** your thinking, and take **intentional actions** that reflect a clearer understanding of yourself in relation to the people and environment you engage with. This is where true **self-transformation** occurs, creating a balanced flow between your **sense of self** and your **sense of feel for self** in the context of real-world experiences.

32. The Process of Applying Brain Care—Self-Care Education.

When you **think through the things you feel**, you're engaging in an inner dialogue that reflects on both **positive and negative emotions**. This reflection enables you to **focus on the experience**, making you more aware of how emotions influence your thoughts. As you begin to **act through your sense of feel for self**, the **receive path** shifts into **response mode**, allowing you to engage with your environment and process the information through a clearer understanding of self.

By choosing to **participate in this process**, you elevate your **awareness**, moving toward a state of **self-directed learning**. This involves recognizing the **changes** that occur as you move between **thought and emotion**, understanding how your **brain and body** co-influence these experiences. In essence, you start to recognize how your **sense, feel, and focus** cycles enhance the receive path's ability to perform, and through this **self-help practice**, you develop greater clarity in how you manage **brain, body, and sense coaction**.

This is where **self-care education** comes into play. The act of **self-care** is intrinsically linked to **brain care**, which is the practice of nurturing your **sense of self** and your **sense of feel for self** by paying attention to the **neurophysics of self**—how your brain, body, and senses interact and influence each other. By understanding and applying **brain care**, you're effectively learning how to integrate **self-technology**—the inherent **technologies of self**—that include your brain, body, and senses working together.

In other words, **self-care education** involves more than just maintaining physical health; it's about recognizing the **dynamic interplay** of your **brain, body, and senses**. The more you practice this, the more you strengthen your understanding of **sense and receive path functions**, enabling you to **improve** how you navigate your emotions, thoughts, and reflections. Ultimately, this journey leads to a more balanced and informed sense of self, empowering you to **actively manage** your brain's role in shaping your overall well-being.

A Progressive Investing Model 36

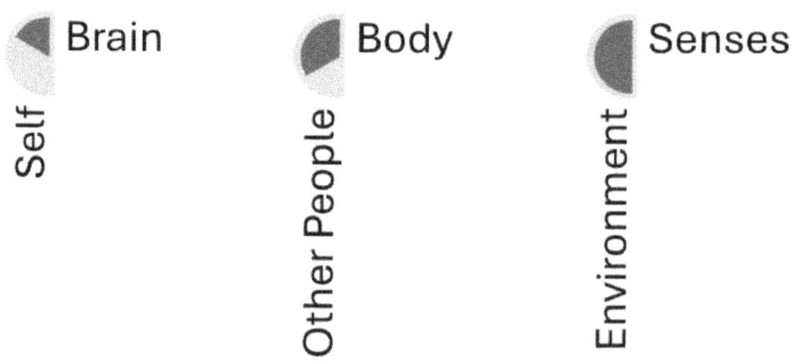

As a **human learning consultant** with over 30 years of experience applying **Human Systems Research**, I've committed to studying **self, other people, and the environment** through a lens that integrates the **brain, body, and sense events**. This work revolves around understanding how individuals can grow by **learning from the experiences** of **contact (self-awareness), interaction (self-connection), and cooperation (neurophysics of self)**. The idea is to shape how we **receive signs of care** from ourselves, from others, and from the environment—or, in many cases, why those signs may be absent.

Human Systems Research offers practical methods for moving through life's interactions more efficiently, by learning to interpret how **contact** affects body language and how it reflects **states of mind**. By understanding how people read and interpret your **body language**, whether as a **positive or negative influence**, you begin to see how your actions affect their willingness to engage with you. This is crucial in human learning, as it is often **mental activity**, not emotional resistance, that drives productive interaction.

At the core of this research is the idea that **self-care** is foundational. The way you present yourself to the world, whether with signs of calm or emotional resistance, directly impacts how others respond. The **crisis of self** emerges when the brain is upset by contact, with **body language** reflecting internal confusion or conflict. As a practitioner, you must observe this, realizing that the other person may not be open to receiving your care without first **moving through self-study** to assess whether they perceive you as a **threat** or ally. This involves communicating with their **brain**, not merely their body, guiding them to feel **safe enough to engage** in a mutual exchange of care.

When working with someone, the **receive path** is where you observe how the brain reflects on the **experiences of contact** and **neural interaction**. This involves listening closely to **noises, sounds, signs, and symbols**, and looking for cues that indicate either **cooperation or resistance**. If cooperation is present, it reflects a willingness to adjust one's **state of mind** and accept your help.

Talking to the brain means helping someone process their **sense and receive path functions**. The focus is on **reading and observing self-interaction**, identifying whether their responses signal **self-correction** or a readiness to accept **care and transformation**. By engaging in this process, we activate **brain talk**, which enables deeper reflection and interaction through **sense and receive path functionality**.

In essence, when we **talk to the brain**, we are guiding people to **organize and express** their experiences in ways that promote understanding and self-growth. The words we use, the conversations we have, and the actions we take all become a form of forward and backward feed between **brain, body, and sense messaging**, paving the way for meaningful transformation.

A Progressive Investing Model 37

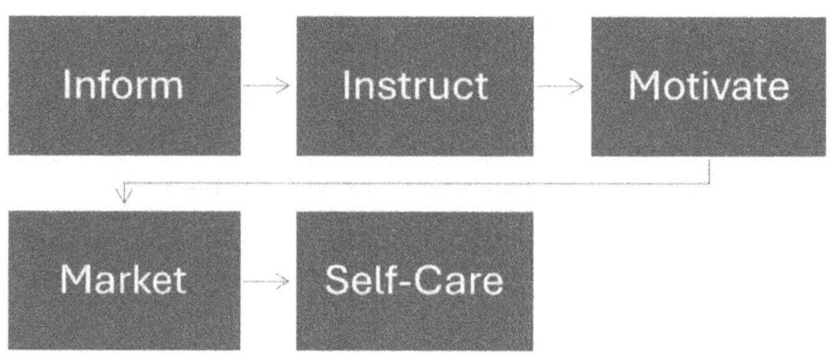

If you cannot move effectively through **contact with written words**, it becomes significantly harder to read and engage with them. This is particularly true when a **sense of feel** for subsequent interaction through the **receive path** is lacking. Without this capacity, it's difficult to generate **backward feed**, the process by which you reflect on and understand your own **signs of care** for physical and neural transitions. This is where **brain, body, and sense research** becomes invaluable. It teaches you not only what **care** looks like but also what **self-care** feels like and why **cooperation** is integral to the process of **self-care education**.

When you can move through someone else's contact and interpret **receive path interaction**, it enables you to read and understand behavior more clearly. This ability becomes a **checkpoint** for gauging the **physics of the body** and the **language of the mind's body**. Such awareness allows you to **protect** your own signs of care by pivoting from mere attempts to inform or instruct, to truly engaging in **self-care technologies**.

For instance, when the **brain leads the body** through a sense of feel for self, the **receive path** responds by guiding how you **read, write, draw, act, perform, and engage** with the brain. Through this, you are practicing the **backward and forward flows** of **thought, reflection, and emotion**—proving to yourself the efficacy of self-care.

You can **feel** how the brain manages information flow through the **sense and receive path loops** and how this, in turn, controls the body's responses. At the same time, you are learning how **brain, body, and sense messaging** creates **energy, action, and feelings** that inform, discipline, and focus yourself through **signs of care** for the experience of the **brain's body**.

In essence, this continuous process of sensing, feeling, and focusing integrates into the practice of **self-research**, and the more you interact with these functions, the better you become at maintaining a balance between **physical and neural transitions**.

33. Thinking with a Sense of Feel for Self-thought, Reflection, and Emotion.

Your body does not think, but it plays a crucial role in receiving sensory information. **Your brain receives sense contact**, enabling it to interact through a **neural sense of feel for self**. The brain utilizes the body to process emotional influences that pass through your **sense of self**, ultimately managing the flow of thought.

The **sense and receive path functions** create thought by channeling **energy, action, and feelings** between your **sense of self and the environment**, and a **sense of feel for self and the brain**, which leads the body's response. This creates a **process loop**, where the brain senses contact and receives interaction, guiding choices to cooperate and participate in **forward and backward feed**.

- **Contact with the body** influences emotion in a backward direction.
- **Interaction with the brain** influences thought and reflection forward.

Through this loop, **sense contact** sets off emotional responses, and **interaction with the brain** generates thoughtful reflection, directing how you navigate experiences.

A Progressive Investing Model 38

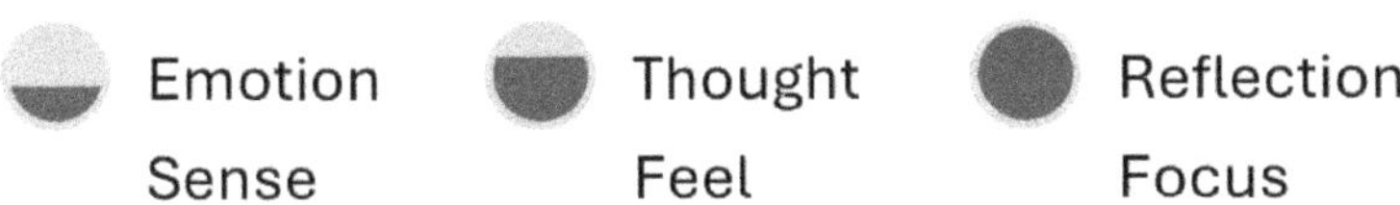

In human systems research, the study of self examines how the **brain, body, and senses** work together to process experiences. When you **sense and receive contact and interaction**, the transformations between a **sense of self** and a **sense of feel for the brain** emerge as critical processes that shape how you think and feel. **Backward feed**—the production of thought, reflection, and emotion—becomes a central concept in understanding how the brain responds to experiences.

Backward Feed: Thought and Reflection

The learning goal is to **accept the transformation** from a **sense of self** to a **sense of feel for self**, with the brain in the lead of the body. This counteracts social and environmental influences that might trigger emotional responses. **Backward feed** informs the sense of self, disciplines the body-mind connection, and **focuses the receive path** to change how you interact going forward. You **think through the things you feel, backward**, which helps you manage your emotions and thoughts.

Study of Self-Emotion, Thought, and Reflection

You think because you feel emotions, and your thinking helps you manage those emotions. The act of thinking simplifies how you navigate your sense of self. In this process, you:

1. **Study Self-Emotion**: Learn how it feels to experience emotions as **brain, body, and sense connections.**

2. **Study Self-Thought**: Understand how it feels to think, and how thoughts connect to the body and senses.

3. **Study Self-Reflection**: Feel what it's like to reflect on experiences and how those reflections affect your brain, body, and sense connections.

Forward Feed: The Inner Voice

Forward feed, or your **inner voice**, is the **mental response** that seeks to solve **information processing problems** from the inside out. It focuses on how you manage the **crisis of self** through your **sense of feel for self** and the brain leading the body. Your states of mind are **manifestations of the exchanges** between the world and your sense of self, and how your **sense of feel for self** uses thought, reflection, and emotion to transform both the self and the world.

In summary, **human systems research** explores how **self-thought, reflection, emotion, and feedback** work together to help you navigate and transform your experiences, using the brain to guide and change your response to both internal and external influences.

The transformation between the **organization of your sense of self**—emotion, thought, and reflection—and your **sense of feel for self** is a critical process in navigating **external influences**. Self-healing, therefore, hinges on **self-learning**, where the **brain acts in the lead of the body** to focus the senses and restore **receive path functions**. This allows you to process and respond to your own **self-research, self-help, and self-discovery** as a **self-care knowledge base**.

Brain-Body Connection and Neuro Physical Awareness

Understanding the **neuro physical awareness** of **brain-body connections** is key to learning how to care for yourself and think through your experiences. When you comprehend how **receive path functions** respond to **physical behaviors** in **sense path transfers**, you open the door to self-improvement. By focusing on the mental actions and physical behaviors involved in these transfers, you can exponentially enhance the brain-body connection.

Learning to Balance Emotion, Thought, and Reflection

The process of self-learning involves **balancing emotion through thought and reflection**. You learn to **manage thought** with reflection, and reflection with emotion, allowing you to accommodate higher levels of self-awareness. This process requires you to:

1. **Sense and feel your inner need to change** in order to elevate your awareness.

2. **Progressively invest in how you learn to care for yourself** by interpreting both physical behaviors and mental actions.

3. Understand how your **sense and receive path functions evolve** as part of this process.

Four Key Areas of Learning Through the Crisis of Self

You are constantly learning how to **navigate the crisis of self** in four fundamental ways:

1. **Learning how you live** through the crisis of self.

2. **Learning how you learn** through the crisis of self.

3. **Learning how you think** through the crisis of self.

4. **Learning how you respond** through the crisis of self.

These stages of learning reveal how the brain and body connect through your **sense of feel** for the **inner-outer process loops**. By focusing on these connections, you gain insight into how to align **self-care** with the evolving challenges of self-awareness, reflection, and emotional balance.

This entire framework emphasizes the importance of self-learning as a way to **restore balance** between mind and body, transforming your ability to respond to external influences and emotional stressors. It is through this continuous **self-discovery** that you develop resilience, awareness, and clarity.

34. When You are in a Self-Crisis, You must be Learnable?

When you feel alone, betrayed, or unappreciated, it's vital to **learn to turn inward** and assess how these emotions impact your **sense of self**. This is where **self-learning** becomes a tool for growth and resilience. You need to understand how your internal reflections translate into **external actions**, affecting not only yourself but also the people around you and the environment.

Self-Analysis Through Engagement

To begin this process, you must **review** your **levels of engagement** in different areas:

1. **Contact:** How do you approach interactions? Do you notice a **withdrawal** or **avoidance** from yourself or others?

2. **Interaction:** Are you open and reciprocal in your relationships, or do you sense a barrier?

3. **Cooperation:** Is there a mutual flow of effort between you and others, or are you doing more or less than your fair share?

4. **Participation:** How active are you in contributing to your environment, and how do others respond to your involvement?

These stages serve as **measuring tools** to examine your **performance** and your **relationships** with others. By doing so, you uncover **patterns** of withdrawal, isolation, or engagement and use this knowledge to improve your **self-awareness**.

Testing Your Sense of Feel for Self

This reflection process helps you test your **sense of feel for self** and whether your brain is truly in the **lead of your body**. This leads to the crucial question: **What does your inner voice say?** Is it constructive, or is it driven by self-doubt and negative emotions?

As this inner voice **transfers to brain talk**, ask yourself:

- **Do I become more mental?** Are you using your thoughts and reflection to navigate through your emotional experience, or are you avoiding them?

- **Do I become more physical?** Do you act out emotionally, or do you channel that energy into productive actions?

- **Do I become more emotional?** Are your feelings dictating your behavior, and how are you responding to those emotions?

Learning Through Self-Discovery

The key is to **learn yourself**—to identify what **drives** you mentally, physically, and emotionally. **Self-discovery** helps you understand your reactions and informs how you can **balance** these areas. When you learn to turn **internal self-talk into constructive brain talk**, you gain control over your responses, turning **self-doubt** and **conflict** into opportunities for growth.

By understanding this dynamic, you can **reshape your interactions** with others and your environment, leading to **improved cooperation, clearer communication**, and ultimately, a **greater sense of purpose and belonging** in your relationships and surroundings.

A Progressive Investing Model 39

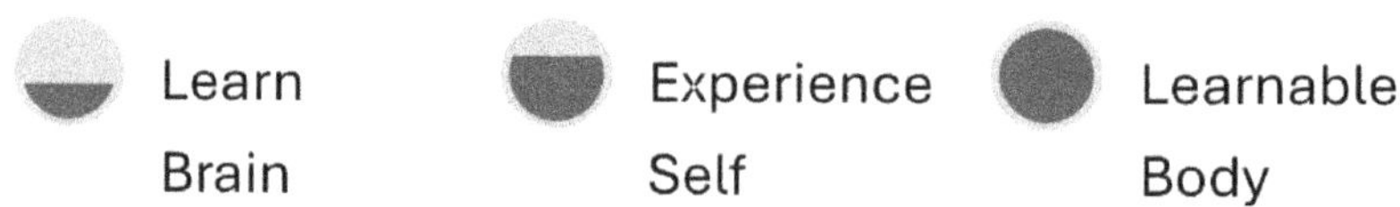

Your idea of being "learnable" from a **human systems science** perspective centers around the profound relationship between the **brain, body**, and the experiences that shape how you interact with the world. Expounding on this allows for greater clarity and brings into focus the idea that **self-learning** is a cyclical process, wherein each interaction—whether from home, school, or work—contributes to the individual's ability to understand themselves, others, and their environment.

By learning the **brain**, you engage in **sense and receive path research**, which highlights how your **sense of self** processes contact and interaction. This is important because learning, from this perspective, is about **solving problems** rooted in the experiences of social and environmental challenges, such as **pain, hurt, and sadness**. Many people face crises, especially when they have not been properly equipped to process the complex experiences of the home, school, or workplace.

Here's how this can be broken down further to enhance understanding:

1. **Acquiring Self-Knowledge:** The ultimate goal is to **acquire self-knowledge** through learning how to navigate the crisis of understanding yourself. In this framework, self-knowledge isn't just abstract; it's about learning how to function when confronted with challenging circumstances. How do you interact with pain, with joy, with uncertainty? The brain leads these efforts by processing the world through **forward feed (thinking and responding).**

2. **Feeling the Need to Care:** One of the key questions in learning the brain is understanding what it feels like to care—or not to care—about the experiences you have. This asks the learner to reflect on their level of **engagement** in their own self-knowledge. If you don't care, how does this affect the way you sense the world, the way you respond to life events?

3. **Self-Research:** Through self-research, you study how your **brain** and **body** respond to experiences. You're not only feeling the emotions but also becoming aware of how your body reacts—how you carry yourself through those experiences. This means learning how to

focus and **acknowledge** the emotions and sensations, which is critical to self-knowledge.

4. **Images of the Body:** Your brain produces **thoughts with reflection** based on the images of the body. This is where your brain acts as a processor, sending feedback about how you're navigating different life experiences. Are you aware of how these experiences are physically affecting you? This reflection helps you see the body and brain as interconnected, shaping the way you respond to **external environmental influences.**

In essence:

- **Being learnable** means learning how to tune into the **feedback loops** between your brain and body.

- It's about engaging in **self-research** to reflect on how the **external world** (social environments) interacts with your internal one.

- The learning process involves **feeling the experience** fully, thinking through those feelings, and then understanding how they shape your sense of self.

A Progressive Investing Model 40

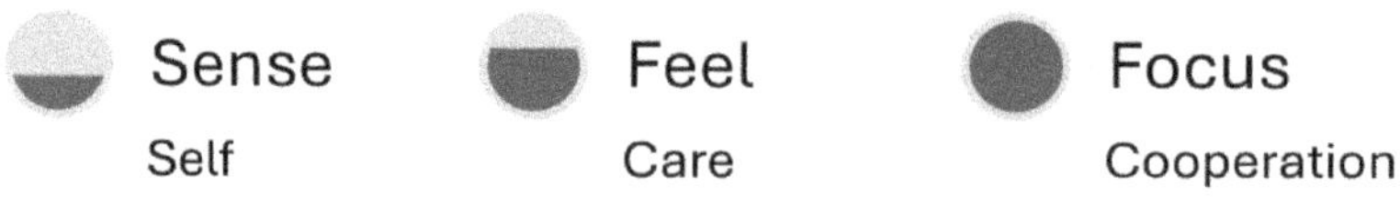

In a **crisis**, the awareness of being in one is often blurred, but asking whether it is your **sense of self** or your **sense of feel for self** that is in crisis can provide valuable clarity. The distinction between these two aspects reveals different layers of **disconnection**:

1. **A crisis of the sense of self:** This occurs when you are unable to interpret or process social contact, often due to a significant life event. It disrupts the way your brain, body, and senses communicate, affecting your interactions with others and your environment. The natural flow of energy, action, and feelings is hindered, making it difficult to exhibit **signs of care—** both for yourself and for others. Without this care, the human system that relies on cooperation and mutual exchanges breaks down.

2. **A crisis of the sense of feel for self**: This reflects a deeper struggle where the emotional connection to your experiences falters. The **receive path**—which involves reflecting on how you feel about social and environmental influences—fails to function properly. In this case, you may be going through the motions but without fully **connecting** to the emotions or thoughts involved. This detachment makes it challenging to learn from or respond to the situation in a meaningful way.

The **key indicator** in both crises is the presence (or absence) of **signs of care**. Signs of care are **tangible expressions** of cooperation—whether it's empathy, understanding, or kindness. These are not just external gestures but internal signals that show your brain and body are working together to navigate the situation.

Signs of Care in a Crisis:

- **For Self:** Are you able to feel concern for your own well-being? Do you treat yourself with kindness, even in the midst of difficulty? If not, the **sense path** (the way you experience contact with the world) may be blocked.

- **For Others:** Are you able to recognize the needs and feelings of those around you? A lack of signs of care for others often indicates a breakdown in the **receive path,** making it hard to connect and cooperate with others.

- **For the Environment**: Are you attuned to the larger context—whether it's the physical environment or the social atmosphere? Without this awareness, you may find it difficult to adapt to changes or process external stimuli.

Self-Experience and Self-Discovery:

A **crisis** often forces a confrontation with questions like *"Who am I?"* and *"What am I becoming?"*. These are not just philosophical queries but **practical realities** of how you function in the world. As you note, your **sense of self**—which includes your **identity, ego, and superego**—is shaped by these moments of social contact. It influences your **personality, attitudes, character**, and **behavior**. However, if there's mental confusion or emotional dissonance, it often stems from a lack of care or regard in how you interact with others or how others interact with you.

In situations where **mental confusion** takes over, it becomes clear that the **sense path** has been compromised. The root cause is often insufficient regard for the **receive path**—a person's ability to absorb and reflect on the contact they've experienced. Without this, the brain and body cannot work in unison, leading to a disjointed **sense of self**.

Your insights, particularly regarding children, are poignant. In your 2006 Progressive Investment Report, you highlighted that **too many children cannot learn**, in part because their **sense**

path has not been given the care it needs to develop. When educators and systems focus purely on **stimulus-response** outcomes without considering how children **feel** the learning process, they neglect the **brain-body connection** that fosters genuine growth. The **sense of self** in these children may be pushed into the background, leaving them unable to fully engage in or absorb the learning process.

When you're in a crisis—whether it's one of self or feel for self—it's critical to **look for signs of care**. These signs indicate that the **brain and body are working together** to process the experience, even under difficult circumstances. Without them, the natural flow of information, energy, and feelings is interrupted, leading to confusion, disconnection, and a lack of progress.

Would you like to explore how these concepts might apply to specific situations or delve further into the ways **signs of care** can be fostered in challenging environments?

Children and adults who have grown up without a connection to how brain, body, and sense messengers send and receive information through sense and receive path participation are less equipped to deal with emotion. The sense path transfers the experience of external contact to the receive path, while the sense of feel for self and the brain creates the learning path for the analysis of self, other people, and the environment. In forward feed, acts of self-research help to learn the sense path, self-discovery helps to learn the receive path, and self-help allows the brain's body to comprehend the flow of energy, action, and feelings.

Brain-body connections raise important questions: Who matters? What matters? Why does it matter? How does it matter? When does it matter? And where does it matter most? Learning how to learn involves understanding how the brain responds to a lack of care and awareness. If children are instructed in ways that don't teach them about the roles and functions of their brain-body connection, they miss out on valuable sense and receive path knowledge.

The transfer of social cognitive experiences to a child's sense of feel for self helps to create brain awareness, something that should not be ignored. Children and adults who grow up unaware of their brain's role in transformation processes often don't respond well to program learning. The brain is designed to change and evolve through the sense of feel for self and the neuro-physics of the brain's body. Struggling with the sense of self means learning how to experience sense and receive path functions by studying how the brain learns, how the body lives, and how the senses feel things.

For someone enduring a crisis of self, the issue is often a lack of connection between the sense of feel for self and the brain. This person may not be able to manage self-thought, self-reflection, or self-emotion. Talking to the brain, rather than the body, is crucial. This involves learning how to engage with self-thought, self-reflection, and self-emotion, ultimately allowing the brain to lead the body through signs of care for self, others, and the environment.

35. A Sense of Your Mind, a Sense of Feel for Your Brain.

Do not hold back. Come to terms with the connection between your brain and body. The body is a physical entity, while the mind serves as a reflective playback device, constantly shaped by environmental influences. The brain, however, is a neural powerhouse, and your body acts as a social cognitive receiver, facilitating mental, physical, and emotional process loops. In simpler terms, the brain is intertwined with the body, and together with the senses, they form what we call the brain's body. This intricate system relies on the sense and receive path functions that transfer information between your sense of self, which is your mind, and your sense of feel for self, which is linked to your brain.

Your sense of mind works in conjunction with your inner voice, while your sense of feel for self is deeply integrated with brain talk. Whether you are reading, writing, drawing, acting, or performing in any capacity, brain talk propels the development of your brain, body, and sense networks, converting self-talk into platforms for personal growth and self-knowledge. These connections shape how you engage with the world and how your inner world communicates outwardly, continuously evolving through mental and physical experiences.

A Progressive Investing Model 41

These elements—energy, action, feelings, emotion, thought, and reflection—are inherent in everything we experience. Each of these components poses unique challenges to either your sense of mind or self, and/or your sense of feel for the brain, which influences how you think and reflect on the experience of self. This area of sense and receive path problem-solving is deeply connected to both the physics of the body and the neuro physics of self. If the flow of information doesn't properly move through your receive path, it becomes much more difficult to reach higher levels of self-awareness through thought and reflection. This creates a backlog in your backward feed, generating a new sense of feel for the experience of self-analysis.

The goal is to enhance your states of mind, pushing beyond static responses to new experiences. Becoming more aware of the self-experience requires a deeper sense of feel for the brain, allowing you to understand how contact feels and improving your capacity to interact. The core objective of your brain-body connection is to sharpen sense and receive path awareness. A critical aspect of self-learning is the mind-body connection to reflective experiences from past thinking. When you shift to a sense of feel for the experience of self, other people, and the environment, you engage deeper levels of focus, enabling clearer thinking and reflection.

When living through a particular state of mind, you might say, "in my mind." When learning through thought and reflection, you may instead think, "let me think this through." This highlights that the mind is a revolving reflective state within the experiences of self, other people, and the environment. To advance your states of mind, you need to introduce new energy, actions, and feelings of thought combined with reflection. This process enriches your perspectives and validates your experience of self, solidifying your brain-body connection. When the brain is in the lead of the body, it allows for the improvement of your states of mind through new stages of receive path awareness, resulting in a synthesis of forward and backward feed.

When you say, "let me think," in the sense of adding more thought, you are preparing the receive path to reconsider the experience. Essentially, you recycle the experience of reflection through self-analysis, asking yourself to think it through. By engaging your sense of feel for the brain, you add more thought to how the information feels in the receive path, allowing you to respond more effectively. This process involves assessing energy, action, and feelings within the experience of contact and interaction, as well as emotion, thought, and reflection. You are reviewing your experience of self in relation to other elements in the situation, like performing a self-check to ensure that you are thinking through different states of mind to become more informed about the information-processing task.

Your mind acts as a state of memory, shaping how you experience and respond to receive path functions. It governs the way your brain, body, and senses communicate. How your brain connects to your body, how your body connects to states of mind, and how your sense of self connects to your sense of feel for self and the brain are all parts of this complex system. Your brain is constantly generating feedback loops, which may include new thoughts and reflections. These feedback loops create the states of mind that you often hold onto as part of your sense of self because the mind's connection to the body manifests in your physical behavior. This is why it's important to feel your way through experiences of self and brain, running receive path checks to ensure that you are processing the information properly. Thinking about how you think involves these receive path experiences of self-reflection.

You engage in thought and reflection not through your mind alone, but through your feelings of self and your brain. The goal is to change your states of mind by improving your sense and receive path performance. The functional goal here is to receive information from your experiences and move through cycles of reprocessing that bring new brain activity into focus. In other words, your sense of feel for the brain drives the shift to deeper levels of thought with reflection as proof of growth. When the brain acts in the lead of the body, it signals changes in your states of mind and reflects new learning.

36. Comprehend the Drive to Survive.

There is another step in your journey: what was normal for you yesterday may no longer seem normal today. You were born with the innate drive to change the world, and that drive fuels your need to learn and adapt to changes in yourself, other people, and the environment around you. This learning process begins within, through your sense of feel for self-experience, and radiates outward as you grow. You must strengthen yourself from the inside out to resist external forces that attempt to dictate how you sense, feel, and focus your brain, body, and sense powers.

The word "live" applies to self. The word "learn" applies to self. The word "think" applies to self. The word "respond" applies to self. These actions are personal, but they also connect deeply to your sense of being. Learning how to live with yourself, learning with yourself, thinking with yourself, and responding with your brain in the lead of your body are essential existential skills. These are the skill sets that define not only how you engage with the world but how you shape and reshape your identity through each experience. Each moment of self-awareness and learning brings you closer to mastering the art of living, thinking, and responding in harmony with your true self.

A Progressive Investing Model 42

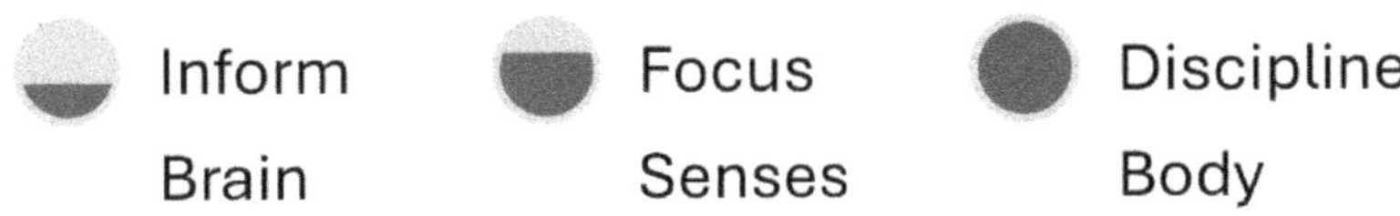

Not everyone has the ability to comprehend the complexity of information flow. To truly understand the experience, one must learn to inform the brain through a sense of feel for self-knowledge. This involves mastering how to inform and manage energy, how to focus thought and feelings, and how to discipline and control actions. The brain utilizes sense and receive path functions to create drives that help you live, learn, think, and respond, ultimately helping you comprehend these experiences across space and time.

At the core of this is the drive to survive the complex layers of self-experience. These experiences—shaped by home, school, neighborhood, and workplace networks—differ in how individuals visualize and understand themselves and others. It is important to ask: Is it your sense of self, or your sense of feel for self, that leads these brain-body experiences? Understanding yourself in relation to others means recognizing how your sense of self and body differ from how your sense of feel for self and brain respond. In essence, brain, body, and sense interplay relies not only on external observations but also on internal feelings to guide responses.

The brain must be in the lead to inform the self, manage energy through the body, and discipline actions. It must focus thought and feelings, both about others and the world, to comprehend the full scope of experiences. This becomes a vital step in developing a more mental approach to life, where the sense of feel for self connects the brain and body, driving interaction and neurophysical energy in a way that requires heightened awareness.

For example, understanding your own self-contact versus another person's interaction can be difficult to perceive. Many struggle with the brain, body, and sense messaging that defines sense and receive path interplay. You may observe someone's actions but not fully understand them due to the unique way they process and respond to information flow. That's why each "Progressive Investing Act" centers around learning to live each day with more focus, discipline, and awareness. The distinction between the sense of the body and the sense of feel for the brain is critical: in the latter, the brain takes the lead.

To "learn" how to live, think, and respond every day, you must also comprehend the impact of human-caused systems like home, school, neighborhood, and workplace networks. These environments are often not designed for your sense of feel for self and the brain to take the lead.

The drive to change the world is innate, but to fulfill it, you must see sense and receive path research as an essential component of self-learning. To live through contact, you need to sense, feel, and focus on the interplay between brain, body, and senses. To learn through interaction, you need to receive, organize, and experience mastery over these connections. To think through cooperation, you must process and respond with care for both self and others. And to respond through participation, you must comprehend the necessity of change in order to perform effectively.

This comprehensive interpretation—that the brain acts in the lead of the body—emphasizes the importance of brain-body neurophysics and body-mind physics. It illustrates how transforming your inner voice into "brain talk" can replace physical, mental, and emotional confusion with clarity and purpose.

37.   Closing Reflections.

As you age into the crisis of self, the choices you've made—both good and bad—begin to echo through your inner voice. Questions arise like, "Why did I do that?" or "What made me act that way?" The key is to allow this negative energy to flow through your sense and receive path functions. By doing so, your brain can take the lead, processing both forward and backward feed to understand your sense of self, inner voice, and states of mind more deeply. Self-learning is the mechanism that detects neurophysical responses in how you sense contact and shift to neurointeraction. It asks if you're resisting or accepting the flow of information, challenging you to assess whether you were truly thinking or just reacting to static states of mind.

When your sense of self is burdened by compounding emotions, it becomes harder to connect with your sense of feel for self. You may struggle to allow your brain to lead, which is necessary for thinking through and overcoming the rigid mindset you find yourself stuck in. Without opening up to reflection—responding with added thought—you might feel worse about your progress instead of better. You may fail to move through the experience and remain in the crisis. However, when your brain takes the lead, your behavior enters a process loop, driving you to seek understanding. You begin searching for ways to think through the influences of pain, resistance, hurt, denial, or sadness—all the emotional labor invested in recovering from self-hurt and sorrow.

This reflection manifests in questions like "What have I done?" You seek to understand, aiming to improve how you transfer energy, actions, and feelings. You analyze the roles your body plays in shaping your states of mind, wanting to reprocess negative energy in a way that brings clarity and relief. By learning to accept responsibility, you connect your brain to your body and senses, checking for changes in how you respond to the world around you. It's not just about reacting—it's about thinking through those mental blocks that previously hindered the flow of information and self-awareness.

This journey proves self-awareness. You move through cycles of forward and backward energy, reflecting on your choices and comprehending them in deeper ways. It's a continuous process of learning and self-analysis, guiding you toward a more profound understanding of yourself.

All the while, you are learning how to cooperate with yourself and the world around you. You start understanding when to go on offense—when to take action—and when to go on defense—when to protect yourself. You navigate brain, body, and sense messaging as proof of your performance, showing signs of care even when you don't feel your best. You may not always feel happy, but you learn how to act through signs of joy. You may not want to laugh, but you learn how to participate and go through the motions. This process is about decoding how you live through the experience of self long enough to transfer that awareness to your sense of feel for self and your brain. You begin to feel good about practicing brain talk. You communicate with your brain, not just your body, reshaping your states of mind and adding more proof that you are progressing in self-learning.

This is why you were born to sense, feel, and focus on brain, body, and sense messaging. It's a process of learning how to receive, process, and respond to both your external sense of self and your internal sense of feel for self with your brain leading the body. In essence, your brain wears your body. This is why you are able to sense contact, receive interaction, feel cooperation, process participation, and focus on self. Your brain is your body—it's your brain's body in action.

At the same time, your body wears your mind. That's why, at times, you appear more physical than mental. You experience yourself as part of the external environment. You may try to live through a sense of self, through body language, moods, and states of mind that reflect physical responses. However, your body doesn't think; it responds to the environmental influences on your brain's body. Your body mind is the external representation of who you are—an effect of cause-and-effect relationships between your brain, your body, and the world around you.

A Progressive Investing Model 44

Brain	Body
☐ Receive	☐ Sense
☐ Process	☐ Feel
☐ Respond	☐ Focus

You write to your brain to transform your inner voice into brain talk, revealing why the brain is housed within your body. This sets up an intricate interplay where the brain leads, the body follows, thought rises, and the mind evolves. This dynamic transforms your sense of self—the body mind—and your sense of feel for self—the brain's body. These transformations are driven by the powers of self-learning, where the brain's leadership over the body influences mental, physical, and emotional harmony. It highlights the importance of aligning brain, body, thought, and mind with the study of sense and receive path research.

Through self-research, you learn how the brain communicates with the body via sense and receive path interplay, striving to balance mental and physical well-being. Brain talk is the process where your inner voice guides your actions and responses to both external and internal stimuli. This research unveils the purpose of self-learning, demonstrating that when the brain leads through your sense of feel for self, you can reprocess rote memories and environmental influences effectively. On the other hand, the crisis of self arises when the body leads the brain, driven by static states of mind and a lack of feel for self, others, and the world.

In the end, this journey of self-learning and sense and receive path awareness allows you to understand how the brain's leadership refines your responses to life's complexities.

ABOUT THE AUTHOR

I AM A HUMAN SYSTEMS SCIENCE THEORIST.
Human systems science theory is the Neuro study of self: and the brain, body, and sense systems as distinct stages of information transfer through sense and receive path channels to assess the flow of energy, action, and feelings. How your brain learns through your inner sense of feel for self. How your body lives through your external sense of self. How your senses think through brain body transformations that describe sense and receive path networks. Such as why the brain receives input, why the senses seek throughput, and why the body responds as output. Hence, I employ a systems approach to human, cognitive, and behavior sciences, i.e., the physics of the body, the mentalism of the brain, and the responses of the senses as the neuro physics of self.

I am Christopher K. Slaton, Ed. D., the voice of Dr. Slaton Live™: Author and producer of Brain's Body Podcast, Education and Science Literature, Brain Talk; Human Systems Science; Human Systems Research and Investigations; Systems Feeling Science; and Chief Executive Officer of the Progressive Investment Group. I developed the Progressive Investing Institute of Focused Learning in 2000 as a laboratory school to study child development through the analysis of brain, body, and sense responses to contact and interaction in home, school, neighborhood, and workplace situations.

Reflective storytelling allows me to write to your brain from a synthesis of more than thirty years of social and emotional knowledge across the applied use of human, cognitive, and behavior science. Through my offerings of education and science literature, I have not only disseminated knowledge but cultivated a bridge between theory and practice, to foster a deeper comprehension of the intricate dynamics that govern our cognitive and sensory compasses of self, brain, and body awareness.

As a practitioner of human systems science, I design Progressive Investing products and services for self-care education: the motivation to learn how to live each day to become more informed through the experience of energy, action, and feelings of emotion, thought, reflection, and feedback.

1. The field of human systems science: the study of brain, body, and sense events to help improve sense and receive path performance.

2. Human systems research, the study of self, other people, and the environment to help improve the contact and interaction of people in their home, school, neighborhood, and workplace as fields of experience.

3. Human Systems Research Investigations, to document the challenges of children who come from a family suffering from substance abuse.

4. Feeling Systems Science, the study of how we feel things, and do we feel the things we feel. "Systems feeling is a new science on how the brain, body, and senses feel things" (Slaton 2010).

5. Brain's Body Learning Systems, the study of (negative or positive) energy, action, and feelings; sense and receive path functions; emotion, thought, reflection; forward and backward feed; and contact, interaction, cooperation, participation, and performance.

6. Brain Talk, the study of language use through the applied use of social and emotional learning as the social neural and science of body mind and brain body interplay through the language of the body and the inner voice of the brain.

7. The general principles of self-talk is the interaction that takes place between your sense of self and your sense of feel for self that converts information processing to forward and backward feed in response to social cognitive space and neuro cognitive experiences.

8. Brain body connections create the capacity and ability to observe, listen, learn, help, and lead through a sense of feel for self.

9. Self-Actualization as a sense of feel for self and the brain, in the lead of the body.